STRIPPED

At the Intersection of Cancer, Culture, and Christ

HEATHER KING

LOYOLAPRESS.
A JESUIT MINISTRY
Chicago

LOYOLAPRESS.
A JESUIT MINISTRY

3441 N. Ashland Avenue
Chicago, Illinois 60657
(800) 621-1008
www.loyolapress.com

Scripture quotations contained herein are from the *New Revised Standard Version Bible: Catholic Edition*, copyright © 1993 and 1989 by the Division of Christian Education of the National Council of the Churches of Christ in the U.S.A. Used by permission. All rights reserved.

Cover art credit: © imagesource/Veer

ISBN-13: 978-0-8294-4262-5   **33614056450884**
ISBN-10: 0-8294-4262-6
Library of Congress Control Number: 2015939790

Printed in the United States of America.

14 15 16 17 18 19 Bang 10 9 8 7 6 5 4 3 2 1

For the lady with the ash-blonde wig

Even the very disease takes on a numinous character.
—C. G. Jung

So the help goes away again without helping.
—One of a series of notes written when, due to tuberculosis of
the larynx, Franz Kafka could no longer speak

*It is characteristic of the true lover that the more he loves, the
more he wants to love.*
—anonymous English mystic, *The Cloud of Unknowing*,
circa 1370

Contents

1

Mercy General

*The century of health, hygiene and contraceptives, miracle drugs
and synthetic foods, is also the century of the concentration camp
and the police state, Hiroshima and the murder story. Nobody
thinks about death, about his own death, as Rilke asked us to do,
because nobody leads a personal life. Collective slaughter is the
fruit of a collectivized way of life.[1]*
—Octavio Paz, from "The Day of the Dead"

At 4:28 on the afternoon of January 3, 2000, I breezed into the lobby
of Mercy General Hospital, just west of downtown L.A. Glancing at
the heart-shaped Mylar balloons, the saccharine greeting cards, the
cheesy arrangements of carnations and baby's breath that spilled from
the gift store, I wondered which would be more depressing: sickness
itself, or having to lie in bed surrounded by that schlock. Then I
clipped a visitor's badge to my arty black sweater, took the elevator to
the second floor, and signed in at the radiology department. Under
"Reason for Visit," I wrote "Mammogram."

I'd purposely taken the last available appointment of the day so
as not to cut into my schedule of writing and errands, and having
squeezed into the previous three hours a trip to Supercuts, a
clothes-buying spree at the Hollywood Goodwill, and a visit to the
library, I found the waiting room eerily still. The only other patient
was an old black woman with bandaged legs, dozing in a wheelchair.

Sickly fluorescent light trickled from the ceiling, a series of air-brushed sunset photos hung from the opposite wall, and beneath a sign that said "Coffee for Patients Only," the hot plate sat empty.

A pleasant young gal with the Virgin of Guadalupe tattooed on her neck made a copy of my insurance card and motioned for me to take a seat. Littered over chairs, strewn across end tables, and overflowing from two plastic holders bolted to the counter were copies of a breast-cancer magazine called *MAMM*. The name made me snicker: years ago my husband, Tim, and I had seen a friend in a stage production of *Little Women*, and he sometimes still called me Marmie. Marm. Are you coming to bed, Marm? I'm going out, Marm; do we need anything at the store? A marmogram.

I picked up a *MAMM*, paged randomly through to a table showing survival statistics, and quickly put the magazine down. I'd had a mammogram every year since I turned forty, seven years before, and though I always acted as if I were performing a civic duty under mild duress, as if the whole thing were a big waste of time because, of course, I was fine, deep down I always approached the appointments with dread. That the payoff for conscientiousness might be disfigurement, suffering, and death seemed so unfair—if so typically one of life's myriad ironies.

I sighed, opened the book I'd brought—Rilke's *Letters to a Young Poet*—and began reading:

> In the deepest places of your heart, acknowledge to yourself whether you would have to die if it were denied [to] you to write. This above all—ask yourself in the stillest hour of your night: *must* I write? Delve into yourself for a deep answer. And if this should be affirmative, if you may meet this earnest question with a strong and simple "I *must*," then build your life according to this necessity; your life even into its most indifferent and slightest hour must[—][2]

"Miss King!" I heard, and looked up to see a pretty, dark-haired woman in a polyester op-art smock.

"Right here," I said, scurrying to grab my purse.

"You were reading," she scolded. "I called your name twice, and you just kept on reading."

"Sorry" I mumbled, thinking, *So is reading a crime now?* My forays into the real world tend to be halting and tentative, and I enjoy them for only limited periods of time—like visits to relatives—until I gratefully retreat again to my books.

I followed the woman down the hall to a windowless cinder-block room, painted pale orange, where she flung me a wrinkled paisley johnny, motioned to an enclosure in the corner, and ordered, "Undress from the waist up."

Behind the makeshift curtain, I draped my black muscle shirt and black bra over a padded chrome chair, donned my johnny, told myself I'd be back in ten minutes, and emerged. Against the far wall hulked a large, insect-like machine of beige metal. I approached gingerly.

"Turn to the right," the technician said, and I instinctively stiffened. I knew exactly what to expect, but that made me more, not less, nervous. She hefted my left breast onto a glass plate; massaged my treasured appendage flat, like a piece of dough whose edges might spring back if released; and electronically lowered a second piece of glass, snatching her fingers away so as to prevent mangling them, and leaving my own flesh compressed in a painful, viselike grip. That a single breast could cover so much ground—squished out flat down there, the thing could have been a pie crust—was mesmerizing.

Then she stepped behind a screen to take a picture, repeated the procedure on the other side, and slapped some labels on the slides. "Hold on; I'm just running these down to the radiologist," she threw over her shoulder, and disappeared down the hall.

I perched on the edge of a plastic chair with my book, but all the people in scrubs and lab coats walking by made concentrating difficult; besides, my johnny was missing a tie and I needed both hands to clutch the front shut. I tried to empty my mind, the way the contemplative mystics I so admired were able to do. But I'd planned on taking a walk afterward, I wanted to be home by six when Tim, an intensive-care nurse, left for his night shift, and after a few minutes I started getting edgy. When the technician finally cruised back in, I was all set to jump up, get dressed, and bolt. And then I heard the nine words that ripped my world apart.

"He wants a second picture of your left breast," she announced, casually loading a new slide.

Adrenaline jolted through my body like electricity; I had a sudden urge to sink to my knees and grab her around the ankles.

"WHY?" I pleaded, in a weirdly loud voice.

"Oh, he thinks he might have seen a little shadow," she said, beckoning me back to the machine with the merest hint of impatience.

I was incapable of responding with any degree of alacrity, as the part of my brain that governs motor skills had been appropriated by a mile-high neon sign pulsing CANCER! CANCER!! CANCER!!! Eventually I shuffled over, weak with fright—it was as if, in the space of seconds, I'd been transformed into an old lady—and robotically removed my arm from the johnny.

"Relax," the tech commanded, trying unsuccessfully to loosen my wooden shoulder: I'm rarely tension free under the best of circumstances, and my body now had all the pliability of someone in rigor mortis. She lowered the glass plate again—"Don't move!"—ran behind the screen to take another picture, and redisappeared down the hall.

I slunk back to the chair and waited, the front of my johnny hanging open (who cared now?), my breaths short and shallow, the way I breathed in nightmares when fleeing from a monster. After a while I realized my heart was beating in rhythm to *Hail Mary, full of grace, the Lord is with thee.* I looked down at my arms.

They were purple with cold, and I'd never noticed how thin my wrists were.

I had never paid much attention to my body, which was perhaps why it was the one area of my life that was characterized by moderation, that wasn't fraught with angst, that radiated health. I hadn't had a drink in twelve years or a cigarette in ten; I exercised, I ate grains and fruits and stout dark greens like kale and rapini; and though I enjoyed clothes and even had a bit of a vain streak, that more or less wrapped up my regimen of personal care. I had no truck with vitamin nuts or vegans, and I considered nutritionists, chiropractors, and acupuncturists to be a bunch of overpaid quacks.

Partly I was too impatient to devote special care to a body that was already sturdy and serviceable; partly I'd deluded myself into thinking I'd been granted good physical health in return for my somewhat fragile emotional health; and partly I'd inherited this attitude from my dyed-in-the-wool Yankee mother, who classified ginger ale as a medicine, considered Novocain a snobbish extravagance and, after the birth of her last child, had gone twenty-nine years without seeing a doctor. I'd always considered Mom slightly over-the-top on the subject, but I had to admit that I, too, had come to treat my body firmly and without emotion, the way you would a dependable tractor. I couldn't remember the last time I'd had so much as a cold, and even during the worst of my drinking, my contact with doctors had been limited to an occasional trip to the ER for strep throat or stitches.

Take a walk, I'd snort to myself when people with vaguely defined conditions such as chronic fatigue syndrome or candida started complaining. In New Hampshire, where I'd been raised, people didn't go to doctors; they worked. They laid brick (as my father had) or dug vegetable gardens or shoveled snow, and though I had always shrunk from such activities as being way too strenuous and time-consuming, I still saw exercise as the surest way of staying healthy, and I still couldn't stomach the rarefied idea of paying money to do it. I walked to the library or bank or grocery store; I took ten-mile hikes in the San Gabriel Mountains; I played tennis for two-hour stretches at a public park in West Hollywood. On summer afternoons, I drove up to the battered courts at Los Angeles Community College, where tufts of grass grew in the cracks of the green clay, and hit old balls against the wall for practice. Working on my backhand in the blazing sun with a discount Big 5 racket, I was a bit proud that I still weighed the same—118—as when I'd played basketball in high school.

Still, lately I'd started to feel protective and slightly sad about my aging body: the blue-green varicose vein that had sprung up on my left calf, the loose skin on my upper arms that quivered when I caught myself off guard in the mirror. And now, shivering in the corner of the mammogram room, I thought wildly, *I'm not old enough to get breast cancer!*

Chronologically, I was middle-aged, but those twenty years of hard-core drinking had cut a deep swath through my emotional growth, and frankly, with my nervous system—no, I was not a good candidate for any illness, especially not cancer. *Cancer*: one of the most horrifying words in the English language, a primal myth, a plague universally loathed and feared. Half an hour ago I'd imagined myself glowing with health. Now I saw myself hairless, shrunken, still wearing this same ill-fitting johnny with the missing tie.

The technician flounced back in, snapped her gum, and said, "Okay, we're all done. You can get dressed."

I rose from my seat, trembling. "So . . . did he say anything?" I asked. "Is it . . ."

"Wanna put your address on here?" she said, pushing a white envelope across the table. "You'll get the results in two weeks."

Before I could ask anything more, she was in the back room dialing her phone. "Yeah, so eight-fifty for the roof, and what about the window frames?" she was saying.

I gave her a little wave when I left, but she never looked up.

On the elevator down I thought, *They must do hundreds of mammograms a week. They must ask for second pictures all the time. A shadow, she said. How bad could a shadow be?* But at the same time I had a vertiginous sense that I had walked through the looking glass into a dream state where my worst fears and reality had finally collided, and when I reached the ground floor, I stopped in at the chapel.

Hospital chapels are like airport terminals: way stations between here and somewhere else; limbos where space and time are suspended; in Celtic spirituality, "thin places," where the boundary between heaven and earth is especially permeable. Votive candles burned on a terraced plastic trolley, an enervated Jesus stared benignly from a mass-produced icon on the front wall, and leftover Christmas music issued from hidden speakers: "O Come, All Ye Faithful," sung by what sounded like a choir of embalmed monks.

The wards above were filled with sick people in their beds, but no splatters of blood, no scalpels and forceps, no birth cries or death rattles intruded here. My own taste ran more to lacerated crucifixes, old wooden carvings of sorrowing saints, Gounod's "Ave Maria" sung by an obscure Italian castrato—but if the hospital had aimed for the blandest common denominator, at least they had aimed.

I thought of the tears that must have been shed in this tiny room, the agonized prayers that had been whispered, the hearts that had cried out in anguish.

I felt the anguish of my own heart: twenty years lost to drinking; a marriage about which I was torn; the recent death of my beloved father; a lifelong sense, in spite of my joy at having found my way to sobriety, Christ, and writing, of searing existential loneliness.

And so in solidarity with all those who had come before and all who would come after, I knelt and prayed: partly lines I had offered up so repeatedly during the past several years they had become like mantras, part naked plea, part suspicion that I was about to face a trial the scope of which I could not begin to imagine. Lord, I offer myself to Thee. . . . I'm afraid, Lord. . . . Pray for us sinners now and at the hour of our death. . . . Lord Jesus Christ, have mercy on me, a sinner. . . . Not now, Lord, I'm not ready. . . . Whatever happens, don't leave me. . . .

After a while my prayer no longer consisted of words. After a while I just knelt there—helpless, flawed, alone. St. John of the Cross wrote, "The Father spoke one Word, which was his Son, and this Word he speaks always in eternal silence, and in silence must it be heard by the soul."[3]

I'm pretty sure I really heard Him that afternoon because after a while, there in that sterile chapel, I experienced a moment of peace such as I never had known before and never have quite known since: a feeling that I might be in for who knew how long a session of sheer unadulterated hell but that somehow, in the end, things would be all right. I'd had moments of peace before, but this moment had a new dimension: this time I knew things would be all right even if I died.

By the door, an oversize scallop shell brimmed with holy water. Leaving, I dipped my fingers in and crossed myself. And all the way through the lobby, past the schlocky gift store and out the door of the hospital, I could hear, *Venite adoremus, venite adoremus, venite adoremus, Dominum.*

Later, when I was going up to the ultrasound lab on the day of my surgery, I was shocked to see the same technician who'd done my mammogram behind the counter in the radiology department, flipping through some files with her long red nails and looking bored. So complete a cutting-off day had that been for me that I could scarcely believe we still inhabited the same world. But, of course, we did not.

She still lived in the land of the well.

I had entered a land in which the only area where I had ever been well had been stripped away.

2

Spiritus contra Spiritum

*It is not true that all reveals God, and it is not true that all
conceals God. But it is at the same time true that He hides
Himself from those who tempt Him, and that He reveals
Himself to those who seek Him.*[4]
—Blaise Pascal

I come from a blue-collar family of, on my father's side, second-generation Irish. We were Democrats, I guess. My father didn't talk politics. He talked the Red Sox, the Patriots, the Celtics. He recited poetry and tended his tomatoes. He was decent, he was kind, he did for his neighbors. He said please and thank you. He was for the underdog. We lived on the coast of New Hampshire, and he was always whipping out his *Boston Globe* at the breakfast table to read us another Mike Barnicle piece about a Little League pitcher with leukemia, or a welfare mother who rode the bus to five different jobs to support her kids.

"Geez, imagine that, the poor soul, out in the cold waiting for the bus," he'd say, shaking his head, and then he'd go off, often out in the bitter cold himself all day, to his job as a bricklayer, by which he supported his own eight kids. "Geez, I hate a guy who blows his own horn," Dad would also say. My mother was a still-waters-run-deep housewife, and we were all wary of, and gave a very wide berth to, "rich people." We did not feel entitled; we felt grateful for what we had. We felt very, very anxious that we might lose it. With black, self-deprecating humor we hid the unspoken fear that perhaps there was not quite room for us at the inn of the "American dream."

I came of age during the sixties and seventies. I had friends who campaigned for McGovern, organized the Clamshell Alliance, and maintained a years-long resistance to the building of the Seabrook (New Hampshire) nuclear power plant. I went along, and certainly agreed, with their stance, and when I got old enough to vote, I voted Democrat—of course Democrat; that was never in question—but I always had my eye on some other realm. I never gave my whole heart to politics. I always felt something was wrong with me, and the world, that no amount of politics could fix.

Since childhood, I'd felt that my job was to bring my family together. *Religion* means "to bind back together," and the impulse to bring everyone around the table, I see now, had been a religious impulse. I was a straight-A student, and the legitimate joy I took in my intelligence was in part a religious impulse. I started drinking at the age of thirteen, and my immediate sense, however false, that alcohol connected me to my deepest self, to God, and to others, was, I believe now, a religious sense.

As misguided as my drinking very quickly became, that I was willing to surrender myself to it so completely sprang from, or generated, a kind of reverse purity that would eventually bring me way beyond caring about reputation, career, money, or any other facet of mainstream existence. That, too, was at bottom a religious impulse.

"You see," Carl Jung observed in a 1961 letter to Bill Wilson, cofounder of Alcoholics Anonymous, "Alcohol in Latin is 'spiritus' and you use the same word for the highest religious experience as well as for the most depraving poison. The helpful formula therefore is: *spiritus contra spiritum*."[5]

I don't quite know how to describe my drinking except that it was desperate even for an alcoholic and that it brought me very, very far from the values with which I was raised. At the University of New Hampshire, earning a BA (in Social Service: my joke was that by the time I graduated, I needed a social worker myself) took me seven years. Financed by a series of cruddy waitressing jobs, I proceeded to hitch-hike across the country, wander around the streets of Boston (where I moved after college) in blackouts, have sex with total strangers, experience degradation, humiliation, poverty. I lived for years in a glorified Skid-Row hotel. I passed out on the landings of the vermin-infested single-room-occupancy tenement where I lived, in locked bathroom stalls in divey bars, and on sidewalks. I came to in strange beds; I came to with bruises, black eyes, gashes; I came to, the sky an indeterminate gray, and called the operator to find out whether it was six at night or six in the morning.

In a last-ditch attempt at normalcy, I applied to law school. For three years I led a double life: student by day, barfly by night. I graduated, cum laude, in more or less of a blackout, increasingly sickened by the knowledge that no way on earth, in my condition, was I ever going to be able to work as a lawyer. I passed the Massachusetts Bar on the first try and went back to waitressing, at a place called Charlie's Beef and Beer, until I came in drunk one night and the cook chased me off with a butcher knife. If it was six in the morning, I fished cockroaches out of glasses of stale beer that tided me over until Sullivan's Tap, the old men's bar in North Station that eventually became my daily hang-out, opened at eight. I lost keys, purses, coats, shoes, my soul.

I was of a certain demographic, in other words, but I had led a very different life than most of my peers. And when I finally sobered up, I found that this had given me not only a certain resident-alien psychic slant, a familiarity with living close to the edge, a deep awareness of my fallenness; it also in a sense had given me less to lose. I don't mean

I didn't care what people thought of me. I cared deeply, and I also very much wanted to contribute. But I was maybe less concerned with appearances, with stepping outside the lines, than I otherwise might have been. I had already stepped outside the lines as far as I could go, in the worst possible way. Nothing could have been more spiritually corrupt, more a missing of the mark, and more mortifying, than the life of an active alcoholic.

And perhaps nothing could have more thoroughly predisposed me for, again, the religious experience of having the obsession to drink removed. One day not drinking had seemed unthinkable, the worst possible punishment; the next day, or rather sometime during the thirty days I spent at a Minnesota rehab in the fall of 1986, I hadn't wanted to drink. I no longer wanted to be anesthetized. I wanted to face the world with a clear eye and an unclouded brain. Call it grace, call it the hand of God, call it a miracle—I had no trouble calling it a miracle—the obsession had been lifted. That for twenty years I had been compelled to drink, and that for the past thirteen years I had not had a drink, was now the central fact of my existence.

I had lived a lie for so long that when I finally came to, I had an almost frantic distaste for, aversion to, cultural lies. As ill-advised as my going to law school had been, in fact, I hadn't chosen the law entirely by accident. I had always wanted to know "how things worked." I was obsessed, when you got right down to it, with how the world worked.

I had thought maybe The Law would show me how things worked. But when, shortly after sobering up, I got married, moved to L.A., passed the California Bar, and started working as a Beverly Hills lawyer, I quickly discovered that the Chief Justice of the Supreme Court didn't anymore know how the world really worked than a Skid-Row drunk; in fact, the Skid-Row drunk knew more: he knew hunger, he knew thirst, he knew that everything depended on a single bottle, a crumb of bread, a kind word.

The culture in which I lived, the air I breathed, told me that smart people believe in science and politics and economics, not in God. Smart people believe in technology. Smart people believe that if only everyone had enough, everything would be all right, which is not only untrue but also ignores the fact that smart people will mostly not share. Smart people, guided by nothing higher than science and politics, will instead try to amass money and power.

The really smart person, it began to dawn on me, will notice that I'm working for people I despise, I'm sleeping with people who don't care about me, my life is a wasteland, and I'm in terrible pain. The smart person wants to be free. The smart person knows she is going to die. The smart person asks, Why am I here? Why do I suffer? What is love?

I had always thought God was for simple people, folks who didn't read or have a sense of humor. But after I'd been sober three or four years, and especially after I started working as a lawyer, I found that I no longer cared whether people thought I was simple or stupid for believing in God.

I wanted to help alleviate the suffering of the world, but how? I wanted to give my whole self, but how? I had always self-consciously joked about my desire to be holy, but I began to see that I did want to be holy. My education had never even acknowledged, much less addressed, such a concern.

As E. F. Schumacher observed in his 1973 countercultural classic *Small Is Beautiful*:

> Education can help us only if it produces "whole men." The truly educated man is not a man who knows a bit of everything, not even the man who knows all the details of all the subjects (if such a thing were possible): the "whole man," in fact, may have little detailed knowledge of facts and theories . . . but he will be truly in touch with the centre. He will not be in doubt about his basic convictions,

about his view on the meaning and purpose of his life. He may not
be able to explain these matters in words, but the conduct of his life
will show a sureness of touch which stems from his inner clarity.[6]

The law didn't begin to give me "inner clarity." The law didn't begin to
answer the questions that haunted me. The law, like much of the rest
of my education, had been largely based on the ability to short-term
memorize. I was good at memorizing and therefore had done well, but
the information I'd memorized had been arbitrary. Arguing motions,
writing briefs, and conducting endless discovery in my cheerless office,
I mused that the information had no value in and of itself. Legal rules
could just as well have been other rules; even language, as beautiful and
useful as language was, could just as well be other words. I wanted to
know the things that didn't have to be memorized—couldn't be memorized—because they were written on the heart.

I began to read books I'd never read before. I began to pray. I began
to go to church on Sunday morning (Tim wasn't much interested):
first to various Protestant churches, because I'd been raised in the Con-
gregational church back in New Hampshire, then to the (especially
ghastly) Unitarian church, then to the Episcopal church. I began to do
something I never thought I'd do: I began to read the Gospels. Nothing much happened on the outside, but a very strange kind of inner
compass came to me completely unbidden and fairly quickly; I simply
knew that in the depths of my soul was the truth, and that truth was
Christ. I was unclear on much else, but I began to get very clear on
what mattered, what master I wanted to serve.

One reason I found Christ so compelling was that he was not
remotely a politician or a lawyer or a social worker. No social worker
would tell a client, "Consider the lilies of the field" (Matthew 6:28).
No lawyer would advise, "Strive first for the kingdom of God and
his righteousness, and all these things will be given to you as well"
(Matthew 6:33). No politician would say, "Whenever you pray, go into

your room and shut the door and pray to your Father who is in secret; and your Father who sees in secret will reward you" (Matthew 6:6).

Like many of my era, I'd tended to think of Christ, if at all, as a gentle, wise, pushover, but the Christ of the Gospels, I discovered to my astonishment, acted with unerring honesty, integrity, intelligence, courage, and above all, love—a kind of love that was always counterintuitive and of an entirely different order than the hearts-and-flowers love of Hallmark cards. The Lamb of God was a figure that no myth had devised: the scapegoat who, himself sinless, had taken upon himself the sins of the world; allowed himself to be delivered into the hands of his enemies; refused to return violence for violence even under brutal, frightful torture; died, and risen, thereby subverting every last earthly power—familial, political, economic, philosophical, scientific, theological, and biological.

Christ had been raised on the Old Testament prophets who, even back then, had observed:

> "In our day we have no ruler, or prophet, or leader,
> no burnt offering, or sacrifice, or oblation, or incense,
> no place to make an offering before you and to find mercy."
>
> —Daniel 3:38

Writing employment-discrimination briefs, hunched over my dank desk, I groped to think of a prince, prophet, or leader in our day, and the only person I could come up with was the unquestionably great Dr. Martin Luther King Jr. Which only proved my point, because MLK had been a preacher, not a politician.

As Clarence Jordan, another visionary Baptist who had established an ecumenical community called the Koinonia Farm during the civil rights struggle of the 1960s, had observed,

> The thing that just burns my heart out is that the Supreme Court is making pagans more Christian than the Bible is making Christians

Christians. The whole integration struggle is being fought not in the household of God but in the buses, depots and around the Woolworth tables in arguments about whether or not we can sit down and eat hamburgers and drink cokes together. We ought to be sitting around Jesus' table drinking wine and eating bread together. . . . The sit-ins never would have been necessary if Christians had been sitting down together in church and at Christ's table all these many years.[7]

I began to see that Catholicism is neither liberal nor conservative. Catholicism is explosively, wildly, anarchically, radical. Catholicism is our hearts, our bowels, our erotic energy, our lives! Look at the Gerard Manley Hopkins poem "Pied Beauty." That "Praise him"[8] at the end is an ejaculation, with the beat, the silence, the lacuna, the gathering in before ejaculation, and it is all the more sublime for having been written by a gay man, a Jesuit priest and severe depressive who offered his suffering, his loneliness, his love, his body, blood, genius, and soul to Christ.

Catholicism is not some timid, rigid, dead set of rules. The whole purpose of the rules is to allow us to explode within them. To be a Catholic is to hover on the edge of orgasm and to consent to continue to hover, indefinitely, in almost unbearable tension, which paradoxically allows us to break out in all kinds of other sublimely interesting, glorious directions and ways. As the writer Alice McDermott notes, "Being Catholic is an act of rebellion. A mad, stubborn, outrageous, nonsensical refusal to be comforted by anything less than the glorious impossibility of the resurrection of the body and life everlasting."[9]

The world says, Play it safe; the follower of Christ thinks, Go for broke. The world says, Let's have an even exchange; the follower of Christ says, Take it all. The worlds says, Send a hundred bucks to the Red Cross; the follower of Christ says, You question how you spend your time and money; you examine your relationships to food, people, work, your body; you make whole, as best you can, the people you've hurt.

You change your life. You come awake into the self you were born to be, and the truly good news is that it turns out not to be any such air-brushed thing as "healthy" or "balanced" or "sane." Was Beethoven "healthy"? Was Van Gogh "sane"? Christ is the über defense against all that is mediocre and banal and sanitized and hygienic and inert and false and shallow and hypocritical and wolf-in-sheep's-clothing and dead, and the über fount of all that is real, beautiful, true, good, astonishing, paradoxical, vital, life-giving, weird, open-your-veins, and funny. He is reality itself: a way of seeing and experiencing the world; the fulfillment of memory, desire, will; the hidden dimension in places, things, and most of all, people.

If Christ had been a cartoon figure, I wouldn't have believed him. If he'd spoken in robotic platitudes, I wouldn't have believed him. If his story had not in the deepest possible way mirrored my own experience of death and unlikely resurrection, I wouldn't have believed him.

Christ was the old men I had sat with at Sullivan's Tap in Boston during the darkest years of my drinking. Christ was Hannah Jelkes in Tennessee Williams's *The Night of the Iguana*, saying, "Nothing human disgusts me unless it's unkind, violent."[10] Christ was the Quay Brothers, stop-motion animators, observing: "It's that little glint, that privileged look into a keyhole, and realizing suddenly that there's this little universe that's probably suffering and barely breathing, but it's pulsating, vibrating, with its own life. That in itself is a metaphor of the universe."[11]

I saw that the call of my heart to write—the call I'd heard since the age of six, the call I thought I'd killed with drinking—was still pulsating, vibrating. I saw I had many wounds and much guilt, and that the wounds and guilt were blocking me. We are all suffering from some gigantic hemorrhaging wound, if not more than one. I think part of the reason people tend to hate the Church with such fervor is that because we are all so wounded, we are compelled, as we are compelled by no other spiritual-religious figure, by Christ. Christ seems like the one Person—as he in fact is—who might understand, who might see what is good and precious in us. And so when the Church fails, as she often does, and perhaps must, the wound is experienced as especially deep.

For my own part, the first time I stumbled into a Catholic Mass, in trembling and fear, I was shocked to see people kneeling. In the middle of Los Angeles, in the middle of the day, people were kneeling. I felt like I'd happened upon a group of folks sitting on the toilet or having sex. Right out there in the open, for anyone who wandered in to see, they were asking for help. They were admitting that they didn't know. They were saying, "I adore you."

Within a year I had quit my job as a lawyer and started to write. Two years after that I was confirmed and took my First Communion at the Church of the Blessed Sacrament in Hollywood.

"The Christian ideal has not been tried and been found wanting," observed G. K. Chesterton. "It has been found difficult; and left untried."[12] "Enter through the narrow gate," Christ said (Matthew 7:13), and you can rig little cardboard dioramas on either side to make it look wider, but it is still going to be narrow. To be a follower of Christ means being certain that we are to love one another as he loved us, and being very uncertain about what that means in any given situation. It means being certain that the light will prevail, and then consenting to walk in almost complete darkness. It means being certain about Christ, and very, very uncertain about ourselves. "The operation of the Church is entirely set up for the sinner," wrote Flannery O'Connor, "which creates much misunderstanding among the smug."[13]

I never thought the Church planned to solicit my vote to see how it should be run. I never thought the Church was going to be one bit more perfect than I was, which, to put it mildly, was not very. I saw what was wrong with the world, with the Church. I had musical sensibilities, aesthetic tastes, homiletic preferences that had been crushed, again and again, to the ground. But my experience had also been this: not once, when my heart had cried out in hunger, loneliness, anguish, or praise, had there not been a copy of the Gospels, a breviary, an altar, a place to kneel, a cross with a body on it, a priest to say Mass and hear my confession. I had never once been encouraged not to die to myself, not to serve the poor, not to continue to quest, seek, and pray.

The struggles, the straying, the brokenness continued. But in the five years since being confirmed, I'd never much focused on what was wrong with the Church. I'd focused on the miracle that she'd taken in a wretch like me.

3

The Vulture's Wing

The increased risk [of contracting breast cancer from birth control pills] is about 3.3 percent per year of use, or 38 percent (relative risk of 1.38) for 10 years of use.[14]
A number of studies suggest that drinking alcoholic beverages, even in moderation, may increase your risk of breast cancer.[15]
Pregnancy also appears to affect breast cancer risk. . . . Women who have never been pregnant seem to be more at risk than women who have a child before 35.[16]
—Dr. Susan Love's Breast Book

I always "knew" I'd get breast cancer. At the chapel in Chimayo, New Mexico, several years before, I'd pocketed a scoop of the supposedly healing dirt and bought a tin milagro: a folk-art charm of a pair of breasts that, back in L.A., I'd nailed to the wall above the bathroom sink in an effort to ward off evil cancer spirits. The once-bright tin had oxidized to a dull brown, and brushing my teeth the morning after my mammogram, I gazed up at my little talisman and thought, *I guess that didn't work.*

One of the reasons I "knew" I'd get cancer was because I'd used birth control pills for five or six years in my early twenties and as soon as I started, I'd gone practically overnight from being almost completely flat chested to having ample, size-C breasts. In one way, nothing could have delighted me more; after that, I always wore the tightest, lowest-cut shirts so as to advertise what I hoped was my extremely alluring cleavage. The women's liberationists maintained that you were supposed to be insulted, but personally I thrilled to the sound of construction workers whistling and calling, "Hey, Baby!" and "Nice rack!" Deep down, though, this precipitous change made me uneasy: wouldn't there be a price to pay for such unexpected bounty? Wasn't there some fundamental wrongness about manipulating nature, some evil that might lie in wait and surface years later?

At the time, I was an undergraduate at the University of New Hampshire, a bucolic campus I escaped every chance I got in search of booze, drugs, and boys. Freshmen were required to live in a dorm, but the moment I became a sophomore, I moved to the nearby blue-collar town of Newmarket and installed myself directly across the street from the local biker bar, at which I basically spent the next six years guzzling pitchers of draft beer, chain-smoking Winstons, and searching in vain for my body-, mind-, and soul mate.

The seventies had been a confusing era. Betty Friedan was braying, "Get out of the kitchen," and I was all for that: from about the age of eighteen on, I was all for getting out of everywhere and heading for the nearest bar. After *The Feminine Mystique*, however, my interest quickly petered out. I dutifully positioned a mirror so as to examine my genitalia (yawn); I wore flannel shirts and construction boots; I plowed through *Sexual Politics* and *The Female Eunuch*, but even then I could never quite get on board.

For one thing, I liked men. I was crazy about my father; two of my closest friends were a tortured alcoholic male poet and a gay, hard-drinking waiter; I'd hitch-hiked across country twice with another bosom tormented guy friend, Michael. Being human, as a gender males naturally had their share of bozos, villains, and creeps, but that hardly seemed a reason to write them all off.

For another, although I'd always had cross-my-heart-and-hope-to-die girlfriends, the notion that I had anything particularly in common with women just because they were women—that I was obligated to regard every female, no matter how boring, venal, or willfully mean, as my "sister"—struck me as at least as coercive and rigid as any of the stereotypes supposedly perpetuated by the legions of chauvinistic men.

Mostly though, even then I knew something was wrong with me that "feminism," if anything, actually exacerbated. Sleeping around, for example, was supposed to be a daring act of empowerment—when my girlfriends and I went out to the bars looking for men, we called it "hunting"—but my own promiscuity arose from the fact that I was lonely and insecure and so blind drunk on any given night I didn't care who I ended up with as long as he was breathing.

Far from liberating me, in fact, indiscriminate sex and the resulting fallout—the betrayals of friends, the rejections and abandonments, abortions—created psychic wounds that would take decades to heal, if those kind of wounds ever fully heal. Many years would pass before the damage was complete, before I understood that sex is a reflection of one's stance toward other people, which is to say one's stance toward the universe, and that when I had sex with a man while totally closed down to the fact that I was a human being, he was a human being, and the two of us might create another human being, I was throwing any number of things out of whack that were going to reverberate way beyond my supposedly private, personal moment.

The real politics of sex, I'd come to see, are that every act, word, and thought affects not only us but also everything and everybody else in the universe. To hold the tension of lust, frustration, and loneliness as a single woman or man, rather than yield to the temptation to use another as object, was to help hold the tension of a sexually and emotionally disordered priest, for example, whose terrible loneliness urged him toward touching a child. To hold the tension of my own lust, frustration, and loneliness as a married woman, and still remain faithful, was to hold the tension of the child who had been touched, and was going to grow up wanting to inappropriately touch someone else: someone younger, someone weaker.

But back in my days at the bars I had not been able to hold any kind of tension at all. Even back then I could feel the dark seeds being planted. Even back then I knew that if I were ever struck down with some dread disease, the illness would implicate my reproductive system, would have something to do with those breasts that had grown too big, too fast.

Twenty-five years later, on the opposite coast, an ex-lawyer, a Catholic convert, and at long last a writer, I had other (though in retrospect, related) things to think about—namely, my vocation/career, my marriage, and my living situation.

Like faith, writing was a matter of life and death to me. Literature had saved my life when I was drinking, and that I now wrote was an honor so profound I could hardly speak of it without wanting to weep. Having taken as my mentor the short story writer and novelist Flannery O'Connor, I was religiously disciplined, perhaps overdisciplined, about my work. I sat down every morning, without fail, and wrote for four hours. I kept a journal. I steadily submitted to magazines, newspapers, small presses, and literary journals. When I wasn't writing, I was reading, or mulling over what I'd written or was about to write, or encouraging others in their writing.

More on my marriage later. Suffice it to say here the fact that I'd gone from making $72,000 a year with benefits as a lawyer to making maybe twelve grand a year with no benefits wasn't helping things go smoothly. I earned seventy-five bucks an hour doing freelance legal research and writing, and zero bucks an hour at creative writing, and that my most fervent wish was to do the absolute minimum of the former and the absolute maximum of the latter will give you a very clear idea of my "business acumen." I didn't expect Tim to support me, but I did want him to support my desire to write, which under the circumstances was asking a lot, perhaps too much.

As for my living situation, I had created the same conditions I had created all my adult life and that seemed to make particular sense as a struggling artist. I, or rather we, had rented a beautiful apartment in a bad neighborhood. For eight years Tim, our cat, Blanche, and I had lived in Koreatown, a "colorful" section of L.A. populated by, in addition to (mostly poor) Koreans (the rich ones lived in Orange County), vast numbers of Mexicans, Salvadorans, Colombians, Nicaraguans, Filipinos, Vietnamese, and the stray fellow Anglo.

Inside the ficus-twined, wrought-iron front gates, our $675-a-month thirties apartment had hardwood floors, crown moldings, and a courtyard filled with roses and gardenias. (I wrote in a tiny room off the kitchen that was essentially the pantry). Outside, I had to chain down the hood of my car because people kept stealing the battery; someone held a gun to Tim's head one night; and I often wondered whether the hordes of ceaselessly shrieking children were a cosmic punchline to the joke that I'd never had any of my own. Our neighbors kicked soccer balls, held barbecues, threw yard sales, sold vegetables from the back of ranchera-blaring panel vans, and worked on their cars, all with about two hundred relatives in tow and shouting at full voice.

Such was the price, or so I told myself, that I was willing to pay for my art. Still, I loved the anonymity of Koreatown, the murmur of foreign languages, being among people without having to communicate with them. Wandering the noisy streets, I could forget my name, my age, where I had come from; I became an invisible stranger in an orphan city. I spent my share of time in hipper, more upscale areas like Larchmont and Silver Lake, but in many ways I felt more at home in my own neighborhood. A mattress with the stuffing coming out in an abandoned lot, a dried-out Christmas tree still blocking the sidewalk in March, a skinny black guy in headphones pushing a shopping cart: that was the poetry that spoke to my soul. That was my L.A.

Sometimes I thought about moving, but perhaps I stayed in the neighborhood just because of the difficulties, because I dimly sensed that living there might put me a tiny bit closer to the people who didn't have a choice in where and how they lived; because in poverty—financial, emotional, spiritual—seemed to lie some essential truth about the world. I had always had a taste for austerity, had always been distrustful of too much comfort, too much ease, and had always been willing to live off the psychological and spiritual grid.

Whatever the case, in time I became almost mesmerized by my inability or unwillingness to leave South Hobart Boulevard. It was as if I were on a kind of obscure mission, as if I were pledged to plumb some mystery, as if, like Jacob, my task was to wrestle with an angel and when dawn broke say, "I will not let you go, unless you bless me" (Genesis 32:26).

The Korean kids next door had driven me crazy for years, stampeding up and down the porch outside the window of the minuscule room where I wrote; a scourge of humanity with their incessant noise. Tim, on the other hand, had not only befriended these adorable pests but also had recently conceived the idea of hosting a pizza party on their behalf. The plans had been made, the children invited—the ringleaders were a pair of siblings named Ben and Emily—and a date decided upon: Saturday night, January 15.

I was cleaning the apartment that afternoon, putting out placemats, hauling the piano bench over to the dining-room table to make two extra seats, when the mail came. One letter bore a return address of Mercy General Hospital. I'd kept myself busy enough so that I hadn't had much time to reflect upon the mammogram, and when I had, I'd pushed the thought uneasily aside. The results had always been normal before; they'd be normal again.

But inside the envelope was a single sheet of paper with a row of boxes down the left-hand side. Only the bottom box was checked, with a big black *X*. And beside the *X*, in capital letters, was the word *ABNORMAL*.

My whole body shut down for a second, and when it returned to life, I saw printed beneath in smaller letters, "Your radiology exam showed an abnormality. Contact your primary-care physician immediately if you haven't done so already."

My first thought was a panicked, *Why would I already have contacted my doctor?* What was I, a mind reader? I pictured a whole flock of women who had learned the rules by osmosis and were way ahead of me; as usual I'd be left panting in the dust, in this case, trying to get an appointment while gigantic tumors bulged from both breasts.

My second thought was, *Couldn't they have chosen a gentler way to break the news? Couldn't they have added, Don't worry: dying takes a while?* Or, as I learned later, *85 percent of the abnormalities found on mammograms are benign?* But no, I was left with that single sinister word—*Abnormal*—and all the possibilities the word conjured.

I sank down on the piano bench, still holding the paper, my mind a jumble of other ugly words: *lump, biopsy, malignant.* I had never before received an abnormal result on a medical test, though in point of fact, I briefly realized, I had hardly ever had any medical tests besides routine blood work and an annual Pap smear.

Tim came back from Domino's a few minutes later carrying a couple of extra large sausages, double cheese. "This oughta hold the little gargoyles," he said, wiping his fingers on one of my nice blue linen napkins.

"Honey, my mammogram came back abnormal," I replied in a strangled voice.

He picked up the report and silently looked it over. "Did you already call the doctor?" he asked.

"NO, I didn't already call the doctor," I almost screamed. "How could I have called the doctor? It's Saturday; he's not even OPEN today."

"Just asking." He leaned down to kiss the top of my head. "Listen, you've got your mother's genes; no cancer cell would dare hang out in you for long. You can call Monday. In the meantime, don't worry about it."

Don't worry, I thought. *Right. I worry when I get good news.*

Again I felt the shadow of death pass over me, the way I had that day in the chapel at Mercy General. I wanted to say, I'm afraid I haven't been good enough, I'm afraid I've disappointed God, I'm afraid I'm not capable of life, I want to go off by myself now and pray! But partly because we are almost always afraid to say what's in our heart, and partly because Tim did not share my beliefs, I knew instinctively not to speak of God.

An hour later the kids came over: Emily, Ben, and two darling itsy-bitsy girls in barrettes and Mickey Mouse sunglasses, all of whom kicked off their shoes, leaving a jumble of shower sandals and neon flip-flops by the door.

After the four of them had minutely examined everything in the apartment, including the drawers of my bedside table, the inside of the piano seat, and the cabinet beneath the kitchen sink, I called,

"Okay, you guys, ready to eat?" and they filed obediently into the dining room.

Tim had ordered two pizzas, thinking one might not be enough, but in spite of their ability to make inhuman amounts of noise, in person the children were tiny and took tiny nibbles, like caterpillars eating leaves. I'd bought Sprite, per Emily's instructions, and poured it over ice in our regular glasses, but their hands were so small it looked like they were trying to hoist tree trunks.

Other than that, dinner went well. Ben picked off rounds of pepperoni and stuck them to his face like scabs. Tim did his imitation of a man pulling a giant worm out of his nose. Emily, I noticed, put her hand over her mouth after every bite.

"Why do you do that?" I asked.

"It's more polite," she said. "So people can't see what you're chewing."

"You ought to try that," I remarked to Tim, who was hysterically laughing with his mouth full of tomatoey crust.

Emily's father worked at a grocery store, she explained: "A long way away on the freeway." Julie's mother worked at home, sewing "little pieces of cloth, like pockets." "All the time, my mother works," little Mink sighed. "Even when we get up in the morning, she's already working."

Everyone had seconds. Over ice cream with chocolate sauce I got them to tell me about their favorite books, kinds of candy, and teachers at school. When a familiar voice sing-songed from next door—Emily and Ben's mother—I ran to the kitchen window and reassuringly exclaimed, "They are good, they are *good!*"

But the whole time part of me was thinking how young they were, how many years they had left, the way that white letter had come floating the four miles from Mercy General to our mailbox, as silently as the wings of a vulture.

4

Dr. Ricketts

I was lucky enough to have health insurance through Tim's job, an HMO policy I'd glanced at once, filed, and never looked at again. Eight years ago we'd chosen a doctor based solely on the fact that he belonged to the medical group of the closest hospital. True, we didn't have to drive very far for appointments, but there the pros pretty much ended.

Ricketts was in his midfifties, with snow-white hair, mottled skin, and a bedside manner that was an unfortunate mixture of bad-taste jokey asides and perpetually rushed rudeness. He ignored my minimal questions, ridiculed my wardrobe—"I see you don't wear nice clothes now that you quit being a lawyer," he once remarked, shooting the cuffs of his monogrammed shirt—and made weirdly inappropriate remarks while performing rectal and vaginal exams: "You're going to feel a pinch now," he'd say, jamming a jelly-coated speculum halfway up to my uterus. "So—have you had anything published lately?"

At least Ricketts remembered what I did for a living: his nursing staff had skipped the course in people skills entirely. Dolores, the neurasthenic whiner who manned the phones, responded to my attempts to converse with a slack-jawed stare; and Myrna, with her shellacked black bun and rhinestone glasses, liked to perform an EKG by slamming into the examining room with the machine, slapping the plastic disks on my goose-pimpled body, taking the readings, ripping off the disks, and slamming out, all without uttering a single word. The three of them had really rolled out the red carpet for my most recent annual checkup. I'd spent an hour and a half in the waiting room, then lain freezing on the examining table for forty-five minutes while they'd celebrated their office Christmas party.

I'd thought once or twice about switching doctors, but Ricketts had steered Tim through several major surgeries, and for the petty annoyances that had composed our health problems as of late, I figured, why bother? If nothing else, he was handy: he knew us well enough by this time so that we'd just describe our hay fever or poison oak over the phone and he'd call in a prescription. Besides, the real reason we stuck with him was that he was a source of good stories because we found his non sequiturs and hopelessly inadequate staff entertaining. The world was harsh. In our household, we took our laughs where we could find them.

Besides—what did I care? I never got sick.

All weekend I kept saying to myself, *At least Ricketts didn't say I had a lump. At least he didn't use that awful word,* LUMP. But when I called the office at 9:00 sharp on Monday morning, his first words were, "Apparently you have a small lump." My heart flipped over and lay there exposed, alone, and squirming. According to Ricketts, the lump was less than half an inch, irregularly shaped, and had been growing for "some months."

"I've ordered a biopsy; 85 percent are benign; call for the authorization Friday," he continued, and signed off. At a minute-and-a-half tops, the conversation was the longest we'd ever had. I had only the vaguest idea of what a biopsy actually was, but I'd known better than to ask my doctor.

Prayer is like practicing the piano or ballet or writing: you have to bring your body for a very long time, in spite of your body's frailties and conflicts and general revolt, and then one day your body is not separate anymore. You've in a sense become the piano or the dance or the word or the prayer. The prayer is in your heart. The prayer *is* your heart.

So my heart surged in prayer, and right away I knew to get on the phone and start making calls to my trusty girlfriends. First I called Iris, who a few weeks before had dramatically announced that she had a life-threatening condition, which later turned out to have been a false-alarm breast-cancer scare. Upon speaking to her, however, I learned that she had never even had an abnormal mammogram, much less a biopsy, but she was still very nice and said that cancer grew really, really slowly, way slower than half an inch a year, and that a friend of hers had had "millions" of biopsies, and they had always turned out negative.

Then I spoke to Ruth, who I recalled had undergone a biopsy several years earlier. I'd been picturing a little session where I'd breeze in, they'd give me a tiny shot of local anesthetic, and I'd breeze out. Ruth was slightly unclear on the details, but she did remember that, no, they had knocked her out. Also, they knew right then whether the lump was cancerous or not: if so, they sent out a sample to be rated as to degree of aggression. Ruth's lump had been filled with liquid (this was what you prayed for), which they had drained and then sent her happily home.

Sylvia, too, had had a biopsy; her lump also had turned out to be a mere cyst, which they had removed—not just drained, but removed—on the spot. "The whole thing was a horror," she kindly reported, "just an all-out *horror*! If they take it out right there, you're okay, but if they bandage you up and send you home—that's when you're in trouble."

Thus began my foray into the strange, mingled-fact-and-fiction universe of often conflicting cancer information. Eventually my friend Kristina faxed over a few pages from the updated version of *Our Bodies, Ourselves*, the feminist all-purpose go-to medical text of the seventies, which reported that with respect to biopsies, the doctor administered a local anesthetic, removed a sample of the lump with a needle, sent the cells out for analysis, and delivered the results a few days later. Several of my friends intimated that they would already have been frantically searching the Internet, but here I (initially) balked. As if a possible medical crisis weren't anxiety producing enough, information gathering had become another civic duty, like mammograms. The only information I wanted at that point was that my lump was benign.

Maybe I was trying to protect myself, and maybe I was hiding my head in the sand. I do know that I could not, under any circumstances, bring myself to try to feel the lump. Every so often my fingers crept to my left breast—Ricketts had said the lump was near the bottom—brushed a tiny patch of skin, and fled back to safety. Knowing that my body harbored an alien, possibly malevolent growth was bad enough. The thought of establishing contact with it made me breathless with terror.

Meanwhile, Tim was showing his true colors: calm, tender, supportive. He did briefly take to calling me "Our Lady of the Rotting Breast," but all in good fun. "I know there's nothing wrong," he kept saying, "but if there is, we'll get the right doctors; we'll see it through together." He displayed nary a trace of the selfish worries that would have plagued me had the tables been turned: What if she can't make money? What if I have to take time out to help?

Like the two other great blessings in my life—sobriety and writing—I had found marriage to be both a gift beyond my wildest imaginings and a crucible in which I was continually forced to work out my most egregious, shameful shortcomings. With his Albert Einstein hair and slightly buck teeth, Tim—a carpenter-turned-nurse—was almost intentionally goofy, a husky, fun-loving puller of lame gags. We'd grown up in neighboring New Hampshire towns, met in high school, and gotten together twenty years later. I'd been newly sober at the time, which meant, in retrospect, that I had not even begun to deal with the massive emotional and sexual baggage from my years in the bars.

Also, though we shared many bonds—food, hiking, humor born of unarticulated pain—our core personalities were very different. I wore my heart on my sleeve; Tim was socially gregarious but emotionally withdrawn. I was optimistically cautious; he was heedless. And while I had never spent so much as a single night in a hospital, Tim had had shoulder surgery, nose surgery and two hip replacements, just in the decade we'd been married.

In fact, Tim was accident prone in a way I found alarming, and I was constantly armchair-psychologist diagnosing him (privately, of course). Time after time we'd have a weekend trip scheduled and Friday night he'd wrench his back or come down with a cold or hit his thumb with a hammer. Out hiking, he viewed "No Trespassing," "Trail Closed Ahead," and "Danger" signs as open invitations to fence-jump and forge on.

As for me, I was an emoter, but I had also learned at a very young age to be self-sufficient. With five younger siblings, I had excelled in school, taken it upon myself to be the glue that held the family together, and as is apparently common in families affected by alcoholism, assigned to myself the role of savior: the one who commanded (okay, craved) attention and yet had—or at least tried to have—no needs. Like my father, I didn't like to bother people, or so I told myself. The truth was that I had an almost berserk fear of rejection, abandonment, and confrontation. The truth was that my self-sufficiency hid a deep neediness and vulnerability.

The upshot was that I tended to think of myself as a victim, I could be terribly passive-aggressive, and my way when in pain was to go into almost complete isolation. I did not like people to help me with my wounds; I would tend my wounds in my way, on my time. No one was more aware than I of my myriad faults: fearful, defensive, overly-sensitive to hurt, a wielder of silent scorn, prone to try to manage and control. My mistake was that instead of taking 100 percent responsibility for my faults, I tended to take 100 percent responsibility for the whole situation.

That I'd become a writer and a Catholic during the course of my marriage shouldn't necessarily have caused a rift in my marriage, but it had. Wanting to give myself unreservedly to my work, I could be testy, impatient, and driven. I said no to a lot of things; I forewent a certain kind of social life, leisure and laxity. In retrospect, I see that I was overly attached to my identity as a writer, that I was unfortunately prone to think that I alone was willing to make sacrifices for my art, and that my willingness to "live in poverty for my art" masked some deeper complexes and conflicts. But at the time, "Store up for yourselves treasures in heaven" (Matthew 6:20), "No one can serve two masters" (Matthew 6:24), and "Love of money is a root of all kinds of evil" (1 Timothy 6:10) were New Testament passages I took very much to heart.

My all-or-nothing thinking led to the conviction that if I just devoted myself wholeheartedly to my work, later I could participate in life fully, later I could "join up," later I'd have more time for Tim. We'd been married by a Justice of the Peace years before my conversion. Even then I'd instinctively known that marriage is a sacrament: ordered outward, consecrated to larger community. I saw now that love is grounded in family: mother, father, if possible, children. I saw now that if you don't have children, you'd better have some other huge shared goal. You have to burn with a white-hot flame toward an endeavor that calls forth all you have—preferably toward all you *both* have.

I burned with a white-hot flame, but was beginning to see that the flame was toward another marriage. Writing was ordering my life toward another realm, a different kind of commitment.

And at the same time, of course, I loved Tim. I loved him, and I felt guilty. Why couldn't I be less afraid? Why couldn't I be more compassionate?

With my cast-iron immune system, I'd always been a little impatient when he got sick. When he came down with a cold during the week I was waiting for my biopsy authorization, though, I felt differently. This time the hacking cough that usually struck me like chalk going the wrong way down a blackboard revealed itself as a cause of concern for him, not me.

"Do you want some Robitussin?" I asked anxiously. "How about a bowl of chicken soup?"

Fear had been my daily companion from as far back as I could remember, and I thought I'd experienced every form of it. But beneath the busyness of my daily life—errands, cooking, writing—a new current had started to run: What if I ever got sick myself?

Ignorant of the health care system as I was, the hateful practice of having to "put in" for an authorization to see anyone besides my primary-care physician came as a rude shock. Ricketts had said the authorization for the biopsy would be ready on Friday. On Thursday, having woken every night that week at three in a cold sweat, I called the office, thinking the approval might have come through a day early. Instead, I learned the office staff hadn't even put in the request yet.

"Oh no," Dolores reported (I swear gladly), "we haven't gotten to that at all. Myrna's sitting all alone in the back room by the computer with just a big stack of those things."

I felt my first stab of panic. Reality hit with full force: Ricketts was an overscheduled automaton; his nurses didn't care whether I lived or died; I was at the mercy of a health-care system in which patients are regarded as irrelevant nuisances. I'd had an abnormal mammogram—why did I need an authorization for a biopsy anyway? Were they actually going to say no?

"Uh, Dolores?" I said. "To tell you the truth, I'm a little anxious over this thing"—I was trying to keep my voice even, but each succeeding phrase came out a little louder and a little higher—"and if I don't get in there, AND FIND OUT WHAT'S GOING ON IN ABOUT TWO MORE DAYS, I'M GOING TO HAVE A FREAKING CORONARY!"

This made about the same impression on Dolores as if I'd remarked that the sun was shining. "Well, I don't know when we'll be able to get to it," she whined. "Myrna"—

I hung up, having no more idea than I had for the past week when the agony of waiting would be relieved.

I often went to monasteries and convents for several days to gather myself, to ponder. In fact, I'd signed up for a retreat at a nearby

Benedictine monastery for the following week. But I was too keyed up at the moment to go on retreat. I was too distracted to engage in any kind of serious reflection.

That afternoon I called and cancelled.

5

Moral Loneliness

The Mass is an extramundane and extratemporal act in which
Christ is sacrificed and then resurrected in the transformed
substances; and this rite of his sacrificial death is not a repetition
of the historical event but the original, unique, and eternal act.
The experience of the Mass is therefore a participation in the
transcendence of life, which overcomes all bounds of space
and time.[17]

—C. G. Jung, *The Archetypes and the Collective Unconscious*

Now I frequented monasteries, but before I converted, I'd barely known the difference between the Old and New Testaments. After a while, though, I'd begun to read the liturgy for Mass (which, being universal, is the same all over the world) each day. I began subscribing to *Magnificat*, a handy little monthly magazine of prayers and reflections. I began to catch fire with the Gospels. I began to feel Christ as a breathing, dynamic presence. I began to see the Crucifixion and Resurrection as the story of our collective psychic journey, of our longing to come awake and be made new.

I discovered Catholicism's poetry, majesty, wild harshness. I discovered that being called to one's highest self required discipline. I discovered prayer, and I discovered that trying to cultivate a technique in this area didn't work for me at all. I paid close attention to Christ's, "And whenever you fast, do not look dismal, like the hypocrites, for they

disfigure their faces so as to show others that they are fasting. Truly I
tell you, they have received their reward" (Matthew 6:16). I took careful note of St. Paul's instruction to pray without ceasing (1 Thessa-
lonians 5:17). I read *The Way of a Pilgrim*, the spiritual journal of a
nineteenth-century wandering Russian mendicant, and adopted as my
own silent prayer the Jesus Prayer: "Lord Jesus Christ, Son of God,
have mercy on me, a sinner."

I discovered one of life's great joys—the Divine Office: daily (almost
hourly, for contemplative monks and nuns) psalms and readings,
feasts, memorials, solemnities; saints and holy days; birth, death, resurrection; the whole cyclical pageant of the liturgical, and human, sea-
sons. Every morning now for years, I'd opened the day by praying
the Office, reflecting a bit on the day's liturgy, and sitting quietly for
twenty minutes or so feeling incoherently happy or confused or overwhelmed: my version of meditation.

I wrote for four or five hours most days, which I considered a vital
part of my practice, if not my existence. I had a spiritual director. I
kept what could be called a spiritual journal. Not as often as I should
have, I examined my conscience at night.

But the heart of my religious life was the Mass, the re-enactment
of the sacrifice that, for a Catholic, is the alpha and omega of the cos-
mos, the sacrament of Sacraments, the act that vanquished death and
thereby established the final, definitive, reign of love: the celebration
of Christ's Real Body and Real Blood.

Mass is divided into two parts: the Liturgy of the Word (readings
from both the Old and New Testaments, always including a reading
from the Gospels) and the Liturgy of the Eucharist (i.e., the Body and
Blood of Christ).

In the Liturgy of the Word, we acknowledge our sins and ask for
God's mercy, offer an opening prayer, and hear the readings (including a responsorial psalm), after which the priest delivers a homily. The

Liturgy of the Eucharist opens (on Sundays) with the Nicene Creed ("I believe in one God, the Father almighty"), and includes Petitionary Prayers, the Preparation of the Altar, the Prayer over the Offerings, the Preface and Eucharistic Prayer, the Lord's Prayer, Sign of Peace, Breaking of the Bread, Communion, Concluding Rite, Blessing, and Dismissal ("Go in peace." "Thanks be to God."). Sunday Mass lasts approximately an hour, daily Mass half an hour.

I often wept during Mass, overcome by emotions I could hardly articulate: by gratitude and reverence and awe; by something of what I imagined Mary had felt when the angel Gabriel announced to her: "The Holy Spirit will come upon you, and the power of the Most High will overshadow you; therefore the child to be born will be holy; he will be called Son of God" (Luke 1:35).

I didn't go to Mass every day, though I sometimes went several times a week and, as the Church asked, always on Sunday—mostly to St. Thomas the Apostle, an Hispanic parish not far from my apartment where I often served as a lector or helped distribute the wine. Other haunts included St. Basil's up on Wilshire Boulevard, with its arms-raised-to-heaven "Our Lady of the Angels" statue, and Immaculate Heart of Mary, a Filipino parish in East Hollywood.

Mass was a way to give thanks, bow to mystery, and connect with the world by offering myself up to this Man who, wholly in tune with God, had mingled with prostitutes, drunks, and tax collectors, looked people in the eye, and told the truth. When Christ came upon a difficult person, he didn't mince words: he said, You're trying to get one over on me; that's not going to do you any good! What's bothering you? When you got overfocused on another person's faults, he said, Whoa, better take a look in the mirror. He consented to live most of his adult life in obscurity, doing the grinding, anonymous work of coming fully spiritually awake, after which he proceeded to live with total integrity, knowing full well that the religious and secular powers would eventually band together and kill him for it.

He was focused on ultimate things every moment of his life, which was why he got exasperated at his disciples, drove the money changers from the temple, and told the Pharisees, You're worried about putting unclean things in from the outside; I'm worried about what's unclean on the inside. He said, Moving a mountain is nothing; the real miracles take place when we tend our own side of the street and let others tend theirs, when we're honest. He loved the lilies of the field and the mustard seed that grew into a bush so large that the birds of the air could nest in its branches; he loved fish grilled over an open fire and good simple bread. He said, in so many words, You have to be willing to endure awkwardness, uncertainty, and pain. You have to love God above all else. That's the way the universe is ordered. That's the only way your joy will be complete.

"Do not think that I have come to bring peace to the earth; I have not come to bring peace, but a sword," Christ had said (Matthew 10:34)—not because he wanted to drive people apart but because to follow Christ means to believe in a version of reality that is very, very different from the "reality" of the world.

To follow Christ means to walk quietly, invisibly, among the people of the world but with your life based on an entirely different order than that of the world; to be willing to accept rejection, scorn, derision, failure, betrayal; to be deeply in touch with your bottomless imperfection, brokenness, woundedness; to consent to any number of extremely unpromising people and situations. But this is where things get interesting.

I mean, we're given all kinds of signs to let us know we're on to Christ, and almost the first sign is that the Way, the Truth and the Life are interesting. You start to change; that's interesting. You forgive someone when you thought forgiving was impossible; that's interesting. The seeming catastrophe transpires, in retrospect, to have helped you along in some way you never could have devised or imagined: that's interesting. You begin to contemplate foregoing a slew of money and security in order to pursue work about which you're passionate: that's interesting.

Christ to me was the most sublime, inexhaustibly exciting subject imaginable, but in the years since I'd joined the Church, I'd discovered that the excitement was not shared by my culture, my demographic, my gender, or even, in many cases, by my fellow Catholics. I had people with whom to walk the spiritual path. I had a faithful family and loyal, generous friends. But I also suffered from an almost unendurable loneliness: what Father Ron Rolheiser—one of my favorite spiritual writers—describes as moral loneliness. He writes:

"Our deepest loneliness is not sexual, but moral. More than we yearn for someone to sleep with sexually and emotionally, we yearn for someone to sleep with morally. What we really want is a soul mate."[18]

6

The Garden at Gethsemane

Those who are well have no need of a physician, but those who are sick; I have come to call not the righteous but sinners.
—Mark 2:17

At last, the authorization for the biopsy came through.

I immediately dialed Mercy General, where a harried woman named Lorena answered, scheduled me for the following Wednesday afternoon, and repeated the magic figure: 85 percent of lumps were benign. She also described the procedure: they laid you facedown on a specially designed table and, as your breast dangled down through a hole—was life sad or what?—stuck in a needle and took out chunks of "tissue." I told her of my friends who'd had cysts, and she said that mine was not a cyst—my spirits sank—because they could tell from the X-rays and they didn't do biopsies on cysts. They did ultrasounds. She called what I had a "mass."

After hanging up, I realized there had been a touch of sympathy in Lorena's voice. This first comforted me, then triggered my native paranoia. If they could tell from the mammogram whether the lump was a cyst or a tumor, they could probably also tell whether the lump was cancerous. They knew, and they made you come in and get butchered anyway, just to make money! Lorena was pleasant enough, but a mere pawn in their game.

The next morning I walked up to St. Basil's on Wilshire Boulevard, as I did three or four times a week, for 8:00 a.m. Mass. I was always happy to be at any Mass, and I was always extra happy to see Father Terry celebrating, as he was that day. Father Terry was a sober alcoholic priest and the drug and alcohol liaison for the archdiocese of L.A. He'd say things in his homilies like, "I don't know about you, but I'm always afraid if I 'let go' one more inch, God's going to take away my health insurance." Or he'd reflect on the self-righteous Pharisee who made a big deal out of praying in public and reflect, "Nope, you don't get extra credit. It's not about getting good marks; it's about being willing to let yourself be broken open with love." The sign of true enlightenment, according to Father Terry, was when you no longer walked around all agonized and tortured with a line of perspiration above your upper lip. The sign of spiritual progress was if crazy people weren't afraid to come up and talk to you.

More than anyone else, Terry had introduced me to a living, breathing Christ who had dwelt—pitched his tent—among us. He talked about sin in terms I understood, not so much as stealing and lying and cheating but as the fear and sense of lack that drove you to do those things in the first place. He talked about a Christ who loved people exactly as they were but also invited them to grow up. He was gentle but not soft. He'd say, "When you come alive with love, you can't find happiness at someone else's expense anymore. When you're truly alive, you're going to look at someone you love and say, 'Well of course I'll give things up for you. Of course I'll die for you!'" And he said it with such good humor, his blue eyes all lit up behind his glasses, that I'd be shaking my head in agreement, nodding and smiling, and then I'd realize what he'd really said, and I'd think, *Die*?

Once he remarked, in his usual half-joking, half-serious way, "Of course you don't want to get too much like Christ, because if you do, you're going to end right up on the cross beside him." And though he wasn't a saint, just human in the best sense of the word (though maybe that is a saint), I knew he pretty much lived up there himself. He stuck by all the pissed-off, crazy drunks nobody else had the patience for. He treated the intellectually challenged to lunch; he counseled the terminally confused; he gave sociopaths a ride home.

He talked about Christ being so fully integrated that when he met a person, he could see straight through to his or her deepest longings and deepest wounds. As in the parable of the woman at the well, for instance, when Christ said, "You are right in saying, 'I have no husband'; for you have had five husbands" (i.e., "You're sleeping around, girl, and it's not really working for ya, is it?") (John 4:17–18). As in the story of the paralytic by the pool, when Christ asked, "Do you want to be well?" (i.e., Or do you want to continue to be a mired-in-self-pity victim?) (John 5:6).

Terry had something of that same quality: the ability to see through to your broken core and, without being co-opted by your secret strategies and schemes, to love you anyway. He'd entered the seminary at the age of fourteen, and he'd been sober for twenty-nine years. Watching the way he conducted himself and treated people, I saw that obedience and discipline and fidelity mean something, that they create in a person—no matter what his or her continuing, possibly terribly bothersome faults—a kind of unshakable core.

Which was why I went to Father Terry's Masses as often as I could. I went to see him raise his robe-clad arms after the entrance antiphon and say, "Let's celebrate the victory of love over death and fear." I went because in the Prayer of the Faithful, along with petitions for the war-torn and the sick, he might throw in, "Let's pray for the people who have a lot of money and three vacation houses and are having a really good time."

Most of all I went to receive the Eucharist from hands I knew: the Body that was at the center of all love, all suffering, all mystery; the Flesh passed from the flesh of this precious friend to mine.

On the big Day of the Biopsy, Tim came with me, trailing behind as I led the way to Radiology. The *MAMM* cover story this month was "The Great Debate: Should Yearly Mammograms Begin at 40 or 50?" All these years I'd been conscientiously submitting myself to a procedure that was supposed to detect breast cancer; upon reading the article, I learned that many doctors were beginning to believe that radiation from mammograms, especially in premenopausal women, could instead cause breast cancer.

Just then, a curvaceous Hispanic gal with long wavy hair approached and introduced herself as Lorena.

"You wanna come, too? C'mon." She motioned generously to Tim and led us down a couple of corridors to a small windowless room. At one end a computer monitor displayed a ghostly blue X-ray of what I assumed was my breast; at the other end hunched a mammogram-type machine, and in the middle was the object that had occupied center stage in my thoughts for the past week: the Table with the Hole. Covered in padded beige plastic, with webbed straps hanging from either side, it conjured photos of the death chamber. The hole, about eight inches across, was near the upper end.

Lorena busied herself with a tray of sharp metal instruments while explaining exactly what a "stereotactic core biopsy" (the procedure I was having) entailed. Too jumpy to take in more than random

words—lidocaine, needle, tissue samples—I fixated instead on the fact
that the pathology report would be ready within forty-eight hours.

Tim, on the other hand, was all ears. Ever since becoming a nurse
and learning how to give shots, he'd been mesmerized by needles. We'd
be lying in bed reading, and suddenly I'd realize he was dreamily fin-
gering one of the veins on the back of my hand and murmuring,
"Mmm . . . I could jab a Hep-Lock in there just like that!"

Lorena brandished the needle they were going to use on me now, a
glint of silver and glass.

"14-gauge," she announced proudly.

"I don't want to look at it!" I said, jerking my head away. "God!"

"14!" Tim whistled. "That's big," and I thought of the spikes the
Romans drove through Christ's hands and feet.

I'd been joking around bravely, but as soon as the doctor walked in,
a rivulet of ice-cold sweat ran down my side. He was a loose, rangy
fellow, about sixty, who smelled of cigarettes, looked like he ate lots
of steak, and had long narrow feet encased in tan wingtips. While I
tried not to hyperventilate, he sat down and recited the same litany of
information that Lorena had. Again, I zeroed in on only one thing: the
results would be ready within forty-eight hours.

After I used the bathroom for the third time—my kidneys were just
slightly overstimulated—the moment finally came. They made Tim
leave, Lorena strapped me face-down on the table, laid a heated blanket over me, and clamped my dangling, defenseless breast between two
cold pieces of glass.

"You're going to feel a little bee sting now, Miss King," the doctor
said, and stuck me with the lidocaine.

When he came at me with the big needle, I started to pray the
Rosary, which, as you may know, consists of three (now four) sets of
Mysteries—watershed episodes in Christ's life and reign—prayed by
means of a series of repetitions through and with his mother Mary. It

was Wednesday, on which the Glorious Mysteries were usually said, but it was the Sorrowful Mysteries—the Scourging at the Pillar, the Crowning with Thorns, the Crucifixion—that came to mind instead as I felt the needle probing inside my breast, heard the whir of their awful machine as it bit out chunks of flesh.

When I opened my eyes, the first thing I saw, sitting on a metal table about three feet away, was a Petri dish full of what looked like blood laced with hunks of chicken fat.

"Man," I felt like saying as I swiveled my head, "couldn't you have put that on the *other* side?" The scene in the opposite direction, however, was no better: an oblong gray canister with "BIOPSY" spelled out on its side in black letters squatted on the floor; the attached clear plastic hose was also clogged with blood.

The doctor and Lorena whispered behind me; I was sure about the sad fact that they'd ascertained at a glance that my "mass" was crawling with malignant cells. As I lay on the table like a stunned haddock, the doctor gave me a little pat me on the back, said, "Good luck! You'll know within forty-eight hours!" and left.

Lorena then bandaged me up, told me I could get dressed, and gave me a paper on aftercare that said under no circumstances should I play sports, drive, or even cook for the rest of the day, a directive I promptly determined to ignore. I'd already wasted the whole afternoon; I wasn't about to lose an evening, too. As soon as we got home, I fired up the cast iron frying pan and sautéed some beets I'd bought at the Hollywood Farmer's Market with garlic and olive oil, sliced a loaf of La Brea Bakery rosemary bread, squeezed lime over a couple of cut-up mangoes.

I had faith, of a sort, but faith does not protect or shield from pain. I had faith, but faith did not relieve me of the terrible, terrible anxiety known by anyone who has ever waited for the results of a cancer biopsy.

Friday afternoon I'll know, I thought all through dinner, the dishes, and several games of cribbage (Tim always won, and I always got slightly pissed).

That night I woke at three, as I did every night now, and lay staring at the ceiling.

"Out of the depths, I cry to you, O Lord," I prayed.

I prayed, "Don't forsake me, Lord."

I thought: *Friday afternoon I'll know. By Friday afternoon, I'll know.*

7

Before I Depart and Am No More

*The cells of the heart which nature built for joy die through
disuse. That small place in the breast which is faith's cramped
quarters remains untenanted for years and decays.*[19]
—Aleksandr Solzhenitsyn, *Cancer Ward*

The biopsy-results mantra continued all through Wednesday night
and Thursday morning, changing in the afternoon to *By this time
tomorrow Ricketts will have called; by this time tomorrow Ricketts will
have called.*

Tim and I had eaten an early dinner, and he was in the bathroom
getting ready for work when, around six, the phone rang. Our phone
was in the minuscule pantry off the kitchen—the room we jokingly
referred to as "the conservatory"—and where, beside the butcher-block
table and shelves of office supplies and food, I also wrote. I ran to
answer, sing-songed "Telemarketer," and picked up.

Instead, a familiar voice said, "Hello, it's Doctor Ricketts." Caught
off-guard—why was he calling today?—I immediately went into semi-
cardiac arrest.

"Is your husband home?" he asked.

That's when I knew.

"He's here, but he's in the shower!" I said. "Why? What is it? Why?
He's here, but he's in the SHOWER!"

"Well, I don't have to do this very often, but I might as well tell you I have some mixed news. Your pathology report showed invasive ductal carcinoma."

Curtains. So I was never going to have the conversation I'd reviewed in my head a thousand times, the one where he said, "False alarm, it was nothing, the lump was benign," and I got to live. Invasive ductal carcinoma: I felt as if I'd left my body and were observing myself from another part of the room, mechanically writing the phrase—"invasive ductal carcinoma"—over and over again, on a yellow Post-it.

"I've requested an authorization for a very good surgeon" he was saying, and "We'll take care of it so it never comes back" (sure), and "Sorry," and then he hung up.

That's mixed? What was the good news? I literally sank to my knees on the floor. Later I realized that this is why people ask if you're sitting down before relaying a piece of devastating news: possibly from a desire to make oneself as small as possible on the theory that the less of you there is, the less pain you'll feel, the body instinctively assumes a self-protective posture by simply collapsing. What flashed before me wasn't my past but my future: years of pain followed by a lingering death or—which was worse?—death within months.

So this is how it happens, I thought, cowering amidst the dusty toolbox, the blue-handled mop, the shelves of orzo and pecans and chopped clams; kneeling on an Oriental carpet that smelled faintly of onion.

Sounds that I had never heard before were issuing from my throat: the hoarse caws of a sick crow. A litany of lines from Scripture welled up from my subconscious: "My eyes are weary with looking upward. O Lord, I am oppressed; be my security!"[20] "They surrounded me like bees; they blazed like a fire of thorns; in the name of the Lord I cut them off!"[21] "Why are you cast down, O my soul, and why are you disquieted within me? Hope in God; for I shall again praise him, my help and my God."[22]

After a minute I realized I had to tell Tim. I stumbled into the bathroom, yanked open the shower door, and wailed, "Honey, I have it."

"Have what?" he cried, his eyes wild, coming out to stand, naked and dripping wet, in the middle of the floor.

"Cancer," I said, "I have CANCER," and he started crying too, and then I was in his arms, the body I knew so well: the broad shoulders, the span of his back.

He offered to call in sick, but his freshly ironed scrubs were all laid out and his unit was having a going-away party for one of the floor nurses that night, so after we'd stood around sobbing for a while and he'd assured me that he'd love me even if I had both breasts cut off, I sniffled, "Nah, I'll be okay, go ahead."

Truly, I wanted to be alone because I was suddenly ravenous for information. I had to start gathering information that instant. Naturally Ricketts had not in any way explained, described, or defined invasive ductal carcinoma, but I didn't need to be an oncologist to know the news wasn't cause for jubilation.

While Tim was getting dressed, I consulted the section from *Our Bodies, Ourselves* I'd decided not to look at unless I had to: the section with information you'd need to know only if your biopsy was positive. "Approximately one-third of the women who get breast cancer eventually die of it,"[23] I read, as the blood drained from my face. I read, skimming, that atypical cells could indicate a range of possible diagnoses ranging from ductal carcinoma in situ, to lobular carcinoma in situ, to invasive.[24]

"Oh my God," I told Tim, extrapolating even as he bent down to kiss me good-bye, "I have the worst kind of cancer you can have."

My usual way of dealing with bad news is to hole up by myself and brood, but instinctively I knew that was not the strategy to employ here. In fact, though I felt like I'd been handed a death sentence, interestingly, I was still myself. My brain was still my brain; my nervous system was still my nervous system; my instincts (surer than I sometimes gave myself credit for) were still my instincts. And my instincts, honed from years of practice, were, as soon as Tim left, to get on the horn and start putting out the word to my sober friends (my form, under the circumstances, of prayer): number one, because I sincerely figured I'd be in the grave within weeks and wanted to say good-bye; and number two, because the sobriety grapevine is the greatest emotional, spiritual, and fact-gathering resource I know.

First, I called my friend Brad, a photographer who wore a T-shirt that read "Tard" and had a bumper sticker on his '72 VW van that said, "I club hippies." "Oh, Heather," he said, "that sucks," and after a reflective pause asked, "Could it have been that time I smoked in your car?"

After we'd followed up with several tasteless mastectomy jokes, he offered to call his friend Clint, a hot-shot surgeon at Cedars-Sinai. Within minutes after hanging up with Brad, Clint rang me. The first thing he said was, "I want you to understand one thing. You're going to be all right. Do you understand? You're going to be all right."

I did not see how he could possibly know that I was going to be all right, but I can't describe how good I felt upon hearing him say it. The next thing he said was that my doctor was a complete and unprofessional jerk for having given me the news over the phone. Finally, he reported that the doctors would probably give me a lumpectomy, six weeks of radiation and, depending on whether the cancer had moved to the lymph nodes, four or five months of chemo. Chemo was one of those concepts so horrible that my mind simply shut down when the word came up, and I decided I would put off thinking in depth about it until much, much later.

Next I called my friend Judy, a landscape architect who had a home in Hancock Park, one of L.A.'s most exclusive neighborhoods, and belonged to the Junior League.

"Oh, Heather," she breathed, "that's terrible. I can't imagine how you must feel. Let me call my friend Lillie from Nevada. She was diagnosed a few years ago, and I know she'll want to talk to you." Ten minutes later, Lillie called. She reported that she had had a virulent strain of breast cancer but that she was now fine, gave me a wealth of websites, book titles, and phone numbers, and briskly but kindly told me to call her at any hour of the day or night.

"The first thing you want to do is get *Dr. Susan Love's Breast Book*," she said. "It's the bible of breast cancer. The second thing you want to do is get a second opinion."

After that I called my brother Ross in Pasadena, who pledged to conduct a blitzkrieg of research. Then I called my sister Meredith in Northampton, Massachusetts. I thought of calling my mother, back in New Hampshire, but with the three-hour time difference she would long ago have been in bed, so I figured I'd wait until morning.

Then I went online and investigated a few random breast-cancer sites. One featured photos of women who had undergone surgery, displaying their naked breasts. You could look at either partial, full, or double mastectomies, but I could only bring myself to view the lumpectomies. One large gal with a blue gingham shirt knotted at her waist had big pendulous breasts; the cancerous one, I was momentarily heartened to observe, looked as if the surgeon had barely taken out anything at all. Then I read the caption: "Now that chemo's over, my hair is growing back great!" I froze, and signed off.

Around eleven o'clock I finally lay down on the living-room couch, stared at the ceiling, and visualized the left side of my chest minus a breast and with a big raw scar instead. The gauze curtains swayed in the breeze; from the balcony bromeliad leaves tapped on the French windows; moonlight shone on the piano, the way the moon shone every night; and I thought, *Oh, let me turn time back, let me have one more week when I didn't know, one more day of innocence, one more care-free hour. . . .*

I thought of the halcyon summer days of my childhood, the dark years in Boston, the day Tim and I had eloped to Nantucket and paid a JP thirty-five bucks to marry us. I thought of the days and nights I had wandered the earth like a pilgrim, the books I had read. I thought of the first time I had entered a Catholic church and seen Christ on the cross above the altar and known to the core of my being that the truth of the world is suffering and the core of the world is love, and that he had come to be with us in our suffering and to show us how to love.

But I hadn't learned how to love yet! I wasn't ready to die! I had so much more growing to do! I'd barely, barely begun!

Falling asleep, I thought of Psalm 39:

> Lord, let me know my end,
>   and what is the measure of my days;
>   let me know how fleeting my life is. . . .
> For I am your passing guest,
>   an alien, like all my forebears.
> Turn your gaze away from me,
>   that I may smile again,
> Before I depart and am no more. (vv. 4, 12–13)

Sometime later I awoke and sprang bolt upright, adrenaline coursing through my veins in a wall of sheer terror: fear amplified to an emotion I barely recognized. Quaking in the dark, I discovered a new prayer—the prayer to draw one more breath without imploding—which, second by second, got me through the rest of the night.

8

Church and State

*Our Western tradition promises that if even a few people find
wholeness, the whole world will be saved. God promised that if
just one righteous man could be found in Sodom and Gomorrah,
those cities would be spared. We can take this out of its historical
context and apply it to our own inner city. Shadow work is
probably the only way of aiding the outer city—and creating a
more balanced world.*[25]

—Robert A. Johnson, *Owning Your Own Shadow*

I often did my best thinking at night. One thing I'd been thinking
about a lot, and pondered throughout this particular night, was the
way the state will do things that are infinitely more corrupt, evil, and
cruel than the Church, yet it's the Church people hate with a burning,
personal hatred. They will despise the state, they will ignore the state,
they will complain about the state, but the burning hatred is saved for
the Church.

Which is interesting because the Church, unlike, say, the U.S. gov-
ernment, does not reign by force. The Church does not come to your
door, arrest you, and deport you to your country of origin if you don't
have a certain set of papers. The Church does not have the power to
stop you in your car, announce they have "probable cause," and search
it. The Church does not reserve the right to examine your belongings,
seize and destroy your belongings, and X-ray you when you board a

plane. The Church does not subpoena you if you fail to show up for Sunday Mass the way the state will subpoena you if you fail to show up for jury duty, or to pay a parking ticket, or to register and insure your car, or to obtain a driver's license if you drive, or to pay into Social Security, or to file your taxes, or to register for the draft and offer yourself up to murder or be murdered for a cause you may find morally, spiritually, and existentially repugnant. The Church does not claim a third of your wages and put you in jail if you refuse to or are unable to pay them.

The (democratic, no less) state does all that. The state keeps eighty thousand prisoners in twenty-four-hour isolation cells: the modern equivalent of medieval dungeons. The state, under cover of night, executes its criminals. If not the state, then the culture, assures that the person of integrity—the artist, the laborer—is more or less forced to live in poverty.

If the Church were responsible for all that, we would rise up as one and say, "This is unconscionable! This is totalitarianism. This is rule by oppression, by force, by brainwashing. This is the evil of religion." Instead we accept, without question, the self-imposed oppression beneath which we live. Yeah, we're grateful the people in power haven't gone completely off the rails and put us in concentration camps, but don't think they wouldn't, given the right circumstance, was my thought. They don't have to, because we willingly enter them and stay there ourselves.

The Church doesn't arrest people: the Church offers the Sacrament of Reconciliation. The state demands a pound of flesh; the Church gives us Christ's Flesh. The state cares nothing for us individually; the Church cares about us only individually. Yet it's the Church people hate. It's the Church that's seen as hypocritical, demanding, merciless, rigid.

The Church hates gay people, the Church-haters say. The Church is anti-sex. The Church is exclusive. The Church doesn't allow everyone to sit at the table. But no one stops you before you take the Eucharist and makes you give an account of yourself. The Church doesn't keep a register, a dossier on anyone. Everyone is welcome. The doors of a Catholic church are open. You could come to Mass every day of your life and be in mortal sin. You could eat Christ's Body and drink Christ's Blood every day of your life and never have been confirmed as a Catholic. No one would say, You have to leave. No one would know (at least in the large city which was my own reference point) but you. The Church is an invitation to come awake, but no one is forced to come awake. The Church operates entirely on the honor system; the Church is our conscience, which is why people hate it—that, and that its individual members and its leaders so often fail to live up to Christ's teachings. But that is no reason to hate Christ; and to hate his Church is to hate Christ.

What's interesting is that the same people who profess to believe that the Host, the wafer, the cracker mean nothing are the very ones who are often the most outraged that it is not willy-nilly available—no questions asked, no preparation, no cognizance of the stupendous significance of the Eucharist—to every taker. People who would not dream of barging into a Buddhist temple or a synagogue or a mosque and demanding to participate, unprepared, untutored, in the highest ritual, are outraged that the Catholic Church, like every other religion, has some kind of minimum requirements preparatory to participating in her highest ritual. The eating of flesh and drinking of blood are so scandalous, so compelling, reverberate so deeply within our psyches and souls, that neutrality may be impossible.

If the Eucharist means nothing, in other words, why would anyone want it? You can't have it both ways. You can't both want the Church to welcome everyone and then, by de-sacramentalizing the Body and

Blood of Christ, remove the one thing that allows it to welcome any-one. Why is the Eucharist such a violent trigger? Why is the Church a perpetual lightning rod? Because deep in our hearts we know. We are compelled. The question hangs eternally in the air: Who do you say that I am? (Mark 8:29).

Another question I had pondered deeply as a lawyer: What did Christ mean when he said, "Give to the emperor the things that are the emperor's, and to God the things that are God's" (Mark 12:17)? The best I could figure was that the follower of Christ sees that the state, whatever its form, is utterly false and corrupt, and walks around it or through it or beyond it, going about his or her business. That the state is corrupt and will always be corrupt is a given. We probably need a state of some kind, and it will always be corrupt. This is one of the myriad places that the edges of Catholicism, which is to say of reality, don't match up.

All you can see is that Christianity is not a social order. All you can see is that the kingdom is not ever going to be at the top—in the state, the nation, in any kind of worldly power. You see that the kingdom is like yeast all through the loaf—in the form of the Christ-centered heart—whatever shape the loaf happens to take: capitalism, Nazism, democracy, socialism. You see that the kingdom of God lies in surren-der, abandonment, humility, loving one another as he loved us, and that abandonment and humility are available to the prisoner in his death row cell, the inmate of the concentration camp, the sub-Saharan African eking out a living with a pickax, the mother in New Jersey, the writer in Missouri, the actor in L.A. You consent to see, as through a glass darkly, and rejoice at the smallest movement of the state toward actually cherishing and protecting its people, and you continue on your journey.

The journey, of course, is to abandon yourself completely, to be transformed by God. The journey is to take the beam out of your own eye, at which point you might be equipped to take the mote out of your neighbor's eye (Matthew 7:5). The impulse is to believe that people will improve if you point out their faults to them. The impulse is to exhort. But to think that the suffering of the world will be alleviated if other people act better is like making your life's work to exhort, Marriage is imperfect! Or People aren't kind! Or You live and then you die! We know that.

"Where are the courageous ones?" the indignant voice perpetually asks. "Where are the saints, the heroes, the martyrs? Where is the real follower of Christ?"

From my bed on the couch, I gazed out over the rooftops of Koreatown. I was just beginning to realize: Oh. I'm supposed to try to be that person myself.

9

Pilgrim Feet

The life of faith is the untiring pursuit of God through all that
disguises and disfigures him and, as it were, destroys and
annihilates him. . . . We would like to know what he has said to
other people, yet we do not listen to what he says to us.[26]
—Jean-Pierre de Caussade, *Abandonment to Divine Providence*

At 5:00 a.m. I rose, went online, and ordered *Dr. Susan Love's Breast Book*. In the first of many instances demonstrating that a little knowledge can be a really bad thing, I also discovered, to my slavering relief, that instead of being a peculiarly grim strain, invasive ductal was a humdrum condition accounting for 75 percent of all breast cancer cases. Not that people didn't die of it left and right—"invasive" meant that the cancer could go outside the cell walls and therefore spread to different parts of your body—but at least doctors saw what I had all the time.

I also learned that if breast cancer was going to spread, the first place the malignant cells generally went was the lymph nodes. Consequently, for diagnostic purposes, surgery routinely included the removal of several lymph nodes from under the arm, a process known as an "axillary dissection." Many women experienced an attendant swelling called lymphedema, which was painful, weakened one's defenses against infection, and often caused permanent loss of range of motion in the arm. As if this weren't bad enough, most of the time the lymph nodes were clear, meaning the patient had undergone all that hell for nothing.

Happily, a delightful doctor from Santa Monica had recently developed a new method of lymph node removal called the sentinel node biopsy. This consisted of injecting the area around the tumor with radioactive dye which, over the course of a couple of hours, traveled the same path to the lymph nodes that cancer cells presumably would. Whichever node the dye stained darkest—the "sentinel" node—was the one most likely to contain malignant cells, if there were any, and accordingly the one the surgeon initially removed: only if the sentinel node contained cancer were the formerly routine ten to fifteen others also removed. In addition to being way less invasive than the old procedure, the new one also had a 99 percent accuracy rate. Thanking my lucky stars I lived in cutting-edge L.A., I made a mental note to ask whether the surgeon I was going to get (on Ricketts' recommendation) was familiar with and performed this newer procedure.

Then I realized, The surgeon *I* was going to get? "You have to be proactive, Mom," I'd counseled my mother the year before when my father had been dying. *Proactive* was the word everyone used in connection with health care these days. Now I realized how cavalier I had been. I could barely remember my name at this point: was I supposed to also canvass doctors, get the names of other patients, call some juggernaut medical board in an effort to locate the best surgeon I could? And if I found him or her, wouldn't the insurance refuse to pay, anyway? Didn't HMOs pay only for hacks?

I could already see that gathering the right information and making the right decisions was going to be nearly as daunting as the cancer itself. At least I had going for me seven years of higher education and a stint as a litigation lawyer, but how did people manage who, say, didn't speak English or read very well? Having one condition to deal with was overwhelming enough; how had my mother navigated the bewildering labyrinth of my father's myriad medical problems: diabetes, congestive heart failure, bad kidneys, ulcerating feet?

One of the women to whom I'd spoken had given me the number of a support hotline in Minnesota called Y-ME. "I found out last night I have breast cancer," I croaked after they'd hooked me up with a counselor.

"And how do you feel about that, dear?" the woman asked.

"I'm scared shitless," I replied.

Calm and encouraging, she gave me the lumpectomy-radiation-chemo spiel, delivered a little pep talk, and reported that she was a twenty-one-year survivor. "Survivor" sounded too plucky and gung ho for me. I did not think of myself so much as having "survived" alcoholism (now I had two diseases with no known cause or cure), as negotiated a delicate, ongoing truce, but I gave the gal my hearty congratulations before ringing off. When Tim arrived home from work, I sat with him while he ate breakfast, filled him in on everything I'd learned so far, and "put him down" (as we called it) for the day.

At nine o'clock I called the cancer centers at UCLA and USC to ask about their second-opinion programs, called my HMO to ask whether they covered second opinions at either or both of those places (they said yes, which later transpired to be a lie), and called Ricketts' office and had them fax over my pathology report. It read:

Diagnosis: Left Breast Mass, Stereotactic Needle Core Biopsy; Invasive Ductal Carcinoma, Moderately Differentiated. Comment: Multiple levels were performed on this biopsy specimen. Because of this, insufficient tissue remains in the block for estrogen receptors, progesterone receptors, and HER-2/neu. Gross [you can say that again!] Description: Received in formalin are multiple cylindrical fragments of yellow-tan soft tissue ranging in length from 1.0 to 0.5 cm and having an average diameter of 0.3 cm. Microscopic Description: Sections examined are of needle core biopsies of breast in which an invasive carcinoma is identified characterized by

malignant cells present in nests and cords with very little gland for-
mation. The nuclei are round to oval. The nuclear membranes are
thickened and many cells contain eosinophilic nucleoli. The mitotic
count is less than 10 mitoses per 10 HPF. The surrounding breast
tissue shows proliferative and non-proliferative fibrocystic changes.

Most of this was unintelligible to me, though one website did offer
that the more well-differentiated the cells, the better. At least mine
were moderately, and not poorly, differentiated, I comforted myself.

Finally, the time came to call my mother. I hated the prospect.
My father, who'd been sick for a long time, had died less than a year
before, and though all eight of us kids had made a tear-jerking, *The-
Waltons*-like rally and spent the last two weeks with him, the experience had been traumatic and draining for all of us. In fact, I'd debated
whether to even tell her about the abnormal mammogram, knowing
she'd worry, and had finally delivered the news only the previous week.

While her phone rang, I thought back to the times I'd been sick as
a child: the pink walls of my bedroom, the galvanized pail beside the
bed, the little round music box with a top of sepia-toned Italian paper
and a crank to be pushed with an index finger.

"I have breast cancer, Mom," I said when she answered.

There was a long pause. Finally: "Oh, Heather."

"I know."

We didn't talk for long, or say much else—but in that moment of
silence, we'd perhaps come closer than we had our whole lives.

Feeling close to people had never been a problem, but actually being
close was not my forte. As far back as I could remember, I had considered "pondering" an essential and vitally important activity. From
my earliest memories, I had been looking for a corner where I could

sit by myself and think. And as an adult, the tension between solitude and community had given rise to constant and recurring conflicts: the vocation of writing versus the vocation of marriage; my love of silence versus the clamor of the world that wanted my time, energy, and presence; my instinctive protection of a psyche I knew was hardwired for solitude versus a world that tends to view the introvert as strange, selfish, and antisocial.

One of the reasons I'd been drawn to Catholicism, in fact, was its long line of contemplative "pilgrims": the Desert Fathers, Brother Lawrence, St. John of the Cross, Carlo Carretto. The compulsion to go off and wander—to connect, to complete oneself, to heal a wound—was as old as man himself, and it certainly had been a continuing theme in my life. I'd hitchhiked coast-to-coast in my younger days, traveled around Europe twice, meandered on foot through every neighborhood, town, and city I'd ever lived in. Tim and I were always taking off for Arizona or Utah or New Mexico to hike and camp. In a way, I'd always been on pilgrimage: always restless, never quite fully inhabiting the place I was in.

One of my favorite "pilgrim" books was *Strannik*, by Russian émigré and activist Catherine de Hueck Doherty. Doherty emphasized that while all are called to pilgrimage, few can or will go. Pilgrimage doesn't necessarily involve traveling, or traveling into the country; the pilgrimage is to our hearts, so the travel can just as well take place in the *poustinia* (a sparse hut or room) of our apartments or into the streets of the city. Wherever we go, we go with bare feet—in spiritual poverty—and because we walk into the fragmented stones and sharp rocks of other people's hearts, our feet get bloody. We're chaste and we're obedient and we fast. We preach the Gospels by living them, and like Christ, we're constantly being called to let things go, to move to another place. We can't be tempted by spiritual riches and gifts, and we make ourselves always available to the people in our lives and those we meet.

Sensing that we're walking the spiritual path, these people ask us about God, and after a while we notice them changing a bit around us. That's what Father Terry did: he was on an invisible pilgrimage, simply going around L.A., talking to and being with and sharing his experience, strength, and hope with other drunks and ex-drunks, and he didn't shut anyone out. People, including me, changed around him.

People didn't change around me, but I did try to make myself available to them. I don't mean I was one of those active, do-gooder types; I was way too self-absorbed and reclusive for that. But just because I was self-absorbed and reclusive, and more to the point, because I was a writer, I'd trained myself to lead a somewhat stringent life. Don't get me wrong—I lacked for nothing. I mean stringent in the sense of doing things that were inconvenient, which to me, was just about any activity that took me away from my writing, involved another person, and didn't further my own personal pleasure, vanity, or mood. Also, to be fair, I craved silence. (I'd once suggested to Tim, "I know—let's have one day a week of total silence!" He'd responded, "How about if we have one day a week where we talk?").

So for me, stringency consisted of participating, of allowing myself to be interrupted in various ways, of wresting myself from the zone of solitude I needed for my writing to talk on the phone, meet for coffee, do small favors, visit people in prisons and hospitals and rehabs, which was time I would have otherwise spent on myself, and which often left me with little nonworking time for myself. Yes, I understood that people worked in coal mines; people hauled rickshaws for eighteen hours a day and slept in the street; people were being beaten and starved and imprisoned. That's exactly why I'd cultivated a life of prayer, reading, reflection, and above all, writing that in one way was all about me, but in another, I hoped, was all about everyone else.

To write in the face of the suffering of the world that seemed to cry out for action; to write when it sometimes seemed my work wasn't bearing fruit; to write because I believed writing, like prayer, to be a good in and of itself, was an ongoing challenge. As the author of *The Cloud of Unknowing*, a spiritual classic written by an anonymous English mystic around 1370, had observed:

> "Just as then Martha complained of Mary her sister, so to this day do actives complain of contemplatives. Wherever you find anyone, man or woman, in any body of people, religious or secular (there are no exceptions), who feel moved by God's grace and guidance to forsake all outward activity and set about living the contemplative life and who, as I say, knows what he is about, his conscience and advisors corroborating, just as soon will you find his brothers, sisters, best friends, and sundry others, who know nothing of his inward urge, or the contemplative life itself, rise up with great complaint, and sharply reprove him, and tell him he is wasting his time. And they will recount all sorts of tales, some false and some true, describing how such men and women who have given themselves up to such a life in the past have fallen. There is never a tale of those who make good."[27]

More and more, though, I saw that with my life of pondering, I had made good. Why we were here, where we were going, how to love our neighbors as ourselves were the most important questions on earth. These were questions I had made it my life's work to ask and that I was now poised to ponder in a whole new way.

I was also being invited to reexamine my deepest wounds—and again, I thought of the wound of my marriage—because those important questions do not arise, nor are they answered, in a vacuum. The questions are always manifested by virtue of, are worked through, and involve the incarnate. "No one comes to the Father except through me," Christ had said (John 14:6). In other words, no one comes awake except through the messy, awkward, lurching, faltering encounter between one suffering human being and another. Love begins, ends, inevitably comes around to, and flourishes or dies in the conflicted, hemorrhaging human heart. I thought of my own hemorrhaging heart, and I thought of Tim's: two emotionally wounded people who, in some poignant stab at wholeness, had gotten married hoping that the other would bring healing.

I had a date to play tennis with my friend Ellen that afternoon, and though to go seemed slightly insane and I was completely exhausted, I felt as if I'd done all I could for the moment, so around one I drove up to Poinsettia Place in West Hollywood anyway. Ellen is smart, funny, a brilliant writer, and one of the gentlest, humblest, most considerate people I know. I gave her the news; we talked over the possible ramifications for a bit, and then she asked if I was sure I wanted to play.

"Yes I am," I said in a small voice. Then I added, "And if you have any decency at all, you'll let me win."

The day was perfect: blue sky, mild breeze. Magenta sweet peas climbed the fence; the coral trees dripped scarlet, sickle-shaped flowers; and out on the court I was thinking, *I might never play tennis again. I might never see the sun again. I might never run around with the mountains in the distance again.* At the same time, I was so overwhelmed that I had ever gotten to experience any of these things at all, so overwrought with gratitude for the miracle of Ellen—this lovely salt-of-the-earth person with whose friendship I'd been blessed—that after the second set I put my racket down, pressed my sweaty, cancerous bosom to hers, and had a good cry behind my Ray-Bans.

Driving back to Koreatown, I realized I'd been exactly right to get some exercise, enjoy the flowers, and remember that other people were my only hope. Almost home, stuck in traffic, I gazed south toward the Art Deco tower of the Wiltern Theater and thought, *Well, one part's over. I will never have to go through the first day after finding out I have cancer again.*

10

Wheel of Suffering

It is solved by walking.
—Attributed to St. Augustine

Now that the floodgates were open, everyone I knew in turn seemed to know at least two or three other women who had, or at one point had had, breast cancer. My friend Ann from Connecticut hooked me up with her friend Claire, a comedy writer who had been diagnosed with cancer in situ (a kind of precancer that has not spread into the surrounding fat cells and is therefore less dangerous than invasive), undergone a preventive mastectomy (!) and was currently recovering from a reconstructive surgery which had involved sewing a flap from her abdomen to her chest (again, !). Rose—mother of four, a nurse, a friend of a friend from back East—had just completed a grueling round of chemo and radiation (her lymph nodes had been involved) and was on a five-year course of a heavy-duty hormone drug called tamoxifen. Nancy, a friend of Father Terry's, had been diagnosed six years ago with both invasive ductal and invasive lobular (more rare than ductal but equally dangerous) and after undergoing a double mastectomy and the strongest chemo available at the time, was alive and well, though still suffering the effects of lymphedema at her job as a supermarket checker.

Perhaps my favorite reaction came from Brenda, an entertainment lawyer with whom I occasionally played tennis and who'd been dealing with breast cancer for the past year.

"Hey, Brenda," I said when I called, "I just got diagnosed myself."

"Oh Gawd, no!" she brayed. "What a royal pain in the ass!"

Suddenly I lived in a world of cancer: every magazine article about cancer, every obituary of someone who had died of cancer. Convinced my own was spreading by the second, every two minutes I felt a pain in my head (possible brain tumor), ribs (lung tumor) or side (ovary tumor).

Within a few days I received *Dr. Susan Love's Breast Book* in the mail, but I found I was able to handle only very small portions at a time. One thing to reflect upon, for instance, was that I'd been innocently harboring alien cells for possibly a decade: "[M]ost cancers have been around eight years before they can be seen on a mammogram and ten years before they can be felt as a lump."[28]

Another piece of information to give me pause was: "Surgery can take care only of the large cancer in the breast itself—if one cell has left the breast and is sitting alone, somewhere else in your body, untouched by the immune system, the most extensive mastectomy in the world won't keep the cancer from returning. That cell will multiply and the cancer will grow."[29]

A handy chart showed how cancer started out with one mutant cell. After a hundred days the one cell had become two; after two hundred days, four; and after eleven years, a lump the size of a walnut had formed, depicted as a nasty-looking blot from which rogue spikes emanated, like a mace.

Maybe the scariest news of all was that when breast cancer metastasized, the cells generally attacked either the liver or the bones. Everyone knew that bone cancer, in particular, meant excruciating pain. I made a big mistake at that point; I read a book by a man named

Robert Lipsyte called *In the Country of Illness*. Robert had recovered nicely from his bout with testicular cancer, but his wife had died of breast cancer that had metastasized to her bones, all described in gory detail, including the spontaneously broken ribs, the wheelchair, and the black gunk running from her nose and mouth at the end. This did not make for restful nights. The terror was too awful to be assuaged even with any number of jokes. No more cancer books for now, I decided.

One thing I knew already, though: I wanted every treatment they had. As horrible as the experience would no doubt be, I was going to demand radiation. I was going to beg for hormone drugs. I was going to make them give me about a year of the strongest chemo they had.

One fringe benefit of a cancer diagnosis, I soon learned, is that people give you presents. A deliveryman brought a bone-white orchid with gold markings and maroon spots from my friend Stephanie; my sister Jeanne sent cards, wildflower seeds, and maple sugar candy from Maine; my artist friend Lindsey mailed an oil she'd painted, all rich yellows and blues, of a Long Island beach. I got lots of books: frescoes of the Chapel of St. Francis of Assisi; Wisława Szymborska poems. My friend Kristina brought over vitamins and decaf green tea. Our downstairs neighbor Emil left a note in the mailbox saying, "Bob [his partner of thirty-five years] and I are here for you, if there's anything we can do." Father Terry left a message on the answering machine: "With you. Praying with you; we'll walk together! Keep open to God's healing."

As much as I appreciated, enjoyed, and desperately needed the support, I soon found that responding to it took up tons of time I would rather have spent writing—that was what I lived for, the hours when

I could forget. Typically, now that I'd blabbed the news to everyone I knew, I wanted to be left alone. Instead, an hour or two every day was taken up with phone conversations, letter writing, and e-mails thanking my friends for their caring and gifts, reassuring them that I was all right.

The only people who seemed entirely unconcerned were my three brothers—Tim, Joe, and Geordie—back in New Hampshire.

One morning I called to talk to my mother and my brother Tim, who was over at the house visiting, answered.

"What's up," he yawned.

"Not much," I snapped, "besides the fact that I have breast cancer."

"WHAT?" he said. "I didn't know you had breast cancer!"

I'd forgotten my mother's penchant for medical euphemism: "low" for suicidally depressed, "spell" for stroke, "spot" for bone-deep gangrenous ulcer. Unable to utter the dread word *tumor*, she'd apparently substituted the word *area*; cancer, in turn, had been reduced to *condition*.

"I was a little bit hurt nobody even called," I let on to Joe when we finally talked later in the week.

"How were we supposed to know?" he said. "The way she talked, whatever you had sounded like something between a mole and a hangnail!"

Caught between the old life and the new, I found that my emotional temperature in those early days vacillated wildly. One minute I'd be cheerfully planning my schedule for the next seven weeks around a course of daily radiation, and the next minute I'd be telling Tim I wanted Fauré's *Requiem* played at my funeral Mass. I teetered between knowing I had a disease that could kill me and the fact that physically,

I'd never felt better. I teetered between the cold, hard world of statistics and the world in which I still needed to sweep the floor and brush my teeth and cook dinner.

And then I teetered down to a place I'd never been before, because after the initial shock had worn off, the next jolt was a deep sense of fragility and loneliness: the realization that, whatever happened, I'd be forever shadowed by the threat of recurrence. I'd recently given Dante's *The Inferno* a close read; now the idea of a dark wood at the midpoint of my life, the descent to a place I'd never known existed, resonated in a new way. And the descent, I quickly saw, was to the fallenness and brokenness of the whole world. I'd always been prone to melancholy, "poor in spirit." Physical illness was a new kind of poverty, and in it, I felt everyone's poverty—not just my own sadness and anguish but the sadness and anguish of everyone who had ever been or was now or would be sick; the knowledge that to survive was no real victory, because someone else wasn't going to.

Then, too, illness was only part of the picture. Suddenly the cruelty and barbarism of the world were borne in upon me with full force: stories of cops shooting innocent men and leaving them to bleed to death, people doing life without parole in nightmarish prisons. A *Los Angeles Times* book review about American lynchings ran a photograph of a black man hanging by his neck, his hands bound, his thighs crossed by whip marks. How to live with the knowledge of that degree of evil (and to admit that you carried such evil within yourself); how to acknowledge and resist at the same time; how to live out your life in love?

One morning, up in Hollywood, I ran into my old friend Fred near the plant nursery where he worked part-time. Fred was a former rodeo rider, long-haul trucker, and Skid Row drunk with a generous heart (even if finding it sometimes took some effort), a hair-trigger temper, and a host of medical complaints: emphysema, a permanently injured ankle, a psyche shattered by the abuse he'd undergone as a child. He'd just gotten out of the hospital, he reported, after a four-day stay for bronchial pneumonia.

"Heather, I gotta get off the cigarettes, I know, I've cut way down," he rasped. "The doctor said 'Listen, pal, I'll tell you straight out, you got a shit pair of lungs; you keep on like this, I give you ten years, tops.' My mother passed away from lung cancer in October, I don't know if you knew that, seventy-two years old."

"I didn't know, Fred," I murmured. "I'm so sorry."

"Plus I found out in the hospital I have hep C, did I tell ya? Maybe five, six days out of the month I feel good. The rest—I'm just not a hundred percent, Heather, but you know me, I'm hangin' in there. Christ, you gotta be grateful, this guy the other night said to me, 'Freddie,' he says, 'most guys that went down as far as you don't make it.' Jesus, that made me feel so good I almost friggin' started cryin'."

We hugged good-bye, and as I watched him limp off in his neatly pressed dungarees and spotless denim jacket, I saw with stabbing clarity that the truth of the world is not in philosophy or science or even theology: the truth of the world is in suffering. The heart of the world is utter, anguished pain. We're hurt, we're angry, we're scared, our hearts are broken, we feel unloved, unseen, unheard. We yearn to belong. We want so badly to believe that we are worth something, that we haven't fallen through the cracks, that our lives are not in vain.

The next morning, walking past a bus stop on 8th Street, I noticed a Mexican guy leading his little boy by the hand, and he, too, had suffering stamped all over his face: the premature age born from years of toil; the sunken eyes, suffused with weariness. They locked with mine for a second, and I gave him a "Yeah, I know" nod of sympathy, but I couldn't tell if he'd caught it or not. All day, I thought of him, thought, *Why should I have things easier than he does, or anyone else?*

That afternoon I took a walk among the stately homes and lushly landscaped lawns of old-money Hancock Park. The rosemary bushes bloomed with tiny purple stars; sycamore leaves stirred in a gentle wind. It was getting dark, with all the things darkness brings in a Los Angeles February: the palm trees turning black against the sky, the smell of jasmine wafting from hedgerows; the sounds—the susurrus of sprinklers, the barking of dogs—muted at dusk.

Behind a lighted window I saw a head bent over a stove, and I suddenly realized that we were all going to die—all the grownups, all the children, all the pets, all the plants. I had never felt so alone, and I had never felt so close to the beating heart of the rest of the world, and when I passed the gate of my favorite mansion and bent my face to the damp pink petals of a Crown-of-Thorns, it came to me with a pang that this was joy.

11

Liminal Space

How dreadful is medicine, dreadful invention of
dreadful people.[30]
—Franz Kafka

If one of the best things about having cancer is getting presents, one of the worst, I soon found, is waiting: waiting for authorizations; waiting to hear from pathologists who may or may not get to your slides by Friday afternoon (and thereby may or may not leave you hanging in suspense all weekend); waiting to hear the meager tidbits of information your doctor feels like dishing out at appointments about which, because you have been kept so completely in the dark about every facet of your case, you fantasize about, anticipate, and dread from every possible angle.

The surgeon Ricketts had recommended was named Staggers. I immediately put in a request for an authorization, called Staggers' office, learned that he performed sentinel node biopsies, and scheduled a tentative appointment for the following week. But just as they had with the biopsy, Ricketts' staff took their time. I ended up having to move the tentative appointment four days ahead—which meant that two weeks after being diagnosed, I still knew nothing more than that I had invasive ductal carcinoma; I still had no documentation other than a one-page pathology report.

I was getting more concerned by the second—about whether the cancer had spread to my lymph nodes and if so, about the possible complications from removing them. Dr. Susan Love wrote: "Unfortunately, not all the complications from your treatment are over when the treatment is. Some of them can occur years later or last for years, even permanently. The major complication, fortunately a fairly uncommon one (10 percent), is swelling of the arm, a condition called lymphedema, which can happen as a result of the removal of lymph nodes. It can be so slight that you notice it only because your rings are gradually feeling too tight on your fingers, or so severe that your arm is huge, even elephantine. . . . It can be temporary or permanent. It can happen immediately, or years after your operation."[31]

I hoped Staggers had a sure hand. A friend of a friend who'd been diagnosed with breast cancer a few years back and also had surgery performed by Staggers couldn't praise him enough (although she, too, now suffered from lymphedema). According to her, he was one of the top surgeons at Mercy General; he had been professional, courteous, thorough. This was wonderful news, but I still couldn't stop thinking about tennis. I am no great tennis player, but perhaps precisely because my game is sandlot and fluky—learned at the age of forty on inner-city municipal courts—the game represented a kind of freedom and fun, a whole way of life almost, that I couldn't bear to think of losing.

Preparing for my appointment, I reviewed my research and wrote out a series of questions on a yellow legal pad. But at the very top of the page I wrote not a question but a statement—I PLAY TENNIS!—shorthand for "Please don't cut some nerve in there and screw things all up so I can't use my arm."

The morning of my appointment, I woke at five-thirty to pitch black, cold, and rain. The previous day I had unfortunately spoken to yet another "survivor," who'd told me about a kind of breast cancer I'd never heard of before called inflammatory, for which, according to her, nothing could be done and from which you died, without fail, within eighteen months. I kept thinking, *Would the surgeon tell me if I had that?*

I kept praying, too. My prayer was never for things to go a certain way but rather a surrender, an opening up, a simple sitting (or standing, or walking, or lying down) and being. Prayer to me was not an activity separate from life, but rather an offering up of every breath, every little thought and act. Prayer was sometimes doing penance for people I resented or judged. If I was feeling particularly hateful toward someone, I'd take the long way home and walk an extra half mile, or go without sugar in my morning coffee—some tiny thing to show myself I was serious when I said I wanted purity of heart.

Tim came with me to the clinic, which was especially helpful as, after painstakingly writing out my questions, I'd forgotten to bring my reading glasses. Also I started feeling very shaky as soon as Staggers called us into his office. He was in his late fifties, debonair, pleasant, even charming, but also a very polished professional who obviously viewed such visits as a matter of numbing routine, had two more people waiting in the reception area, and did not intend to let the appointment last a single second more than was absolutely necessary.

"You understand you have breast cancer, don't you?" he began.

"Yes, I do," I replied, thinking, *Duh!! What do you think I've been obsessed with every waking and sleeping moment for the last three weeks?*

"Now you're going to need some surgery—" he continued.

"I play tennis!" I blurted.

Over the course of my ordeal I would often experience this same cognitive dissonance while talking to doctors. They'd be nattering away about estrogen inhibition, and I'd be looking at their faces, long-ing to report, "I was holding my father's hand when he died." Or they'd be going on about how not to eat or drink for twelve hours, and I'd have to hold myself back from asking, "Have you ever noticed that people with Down syndrome always say hi back, that the less 'smart' the person, the more likely he or she is to acknowledge you as a fellow human being?"

He closed his eyes, as if counting to ten, then opened them and asked, "Are you right-handed or left-handed?"

"Right, but I have a two-handed backhand."

He shrugged, as if to say, *Come, come now, this is no time for trifles: if the knife slips, the knife slips.*

"Your lump was just under a centimeter," he went on (newly branded on my brain was the fact that a centimeter is .39 inches), "so as things appear now, you're in Stage 1. That means you have a choice. You can have a mastectomy without radiation or a lumpectomy with radiation. I don't have a recommendation one way or the other. They've been demonstrated to be equally effective."

I didn't have inflammatory breast cancer! My cells weren't replicat-ing at some outlandishly unheard-of rate! I wasn't going to have to have a mastectomy; I wasn't going to have a mastectomy!

"I don't even have to think about that," I breathed. "Lumpectomy with radiation!"

Not until later did I realize that he had said nothing about what radiation actually is, the risks entailed, or how, if at all, my chances of survival would be improved. Nor did he mention how much of my breast he was going to cut out or what I might expect it to look like afterward. The lumpectomy diagrams in the books tended to portray a pie with a slice taken out—a gruesome prospect—but to inquire under the circumstances somehow seemed churlish. As with the possibility of a severed nerve, the unspoken assumption was that, whatever the postsurgical deficits, they were the price one paid—was in fact thrilled to pay—for a stab at prolonged life.

"What kind of anesthesia do you use?" I asked, checking off another question on my legal pad.

"You can be knocked out completely if you want. Or we can put you in a twilight state where you're technically awake but you won't know where you are, won't care where you are, and won't remember where you are," he said.

"I used to have sex with people in that condition," I offered, guffawing loudly at my own joke (the doctor of course never broke a smile).

Between my questions and the minimal information he offered, we fleshed out the rest of the sentinel node biopsy scenario. While I was on the table, a pathologist would examine samples of the sentinel node. If the node was cancerous, Staggers would proceed to remove ten to twenty more nodes and probably keep me in the hospital overnight. If not, he'd sew me up and send me home.

The kicker, though, was this: the slides were sent out for further analysis, and 15 percent of the time the sentinel node turned out to have been malignant after all. If that happened, not only would my hopes for clear lymph nodes have been dashed, I'd also have to come back, undergo a second surgery, and incur the risk of cut nerves and lymphedema anyway. *Waiting for that news should be a fun three days*, I thought.

All other things being equal, I like to make people happy. I'm glad, eager even to participate. I'm not an agitator. I'm not averse to following the rules, but obedience—"to listen carefully"—is not necessarily synonymous with following the rules. "Do what the doctors tell you, and how they tell you," an acquaintance had recently advised. Which may be sound, commonsense advice as far as it goes, but the SS guards had taken that advice.

I sensed I was poised to consider "the rules" in a new light. I sensed I was moving into what Franciscan priest Richard Rohr calls "liminal space":

> The edge of things is a liminal space. The edge is a holy place, or as the Celts called it, "a thin place" and you have to be taught how to live there. To take your position on the spiritual edge of things is to learn how to move safely in and out, back and forth, across and return. It is a prophetic position, not a rebellious or antisocial one. When you live on the edge of anything with respect and honor, you are in a very auspicious position. . . . To live on the edge of the inside is different than being an insider. Yes, you have learned the rules and you understand and honor the system as far as it goes, but you do not need to protect it, defend it, or promote it. [You can] love both the inside and the outside . . . and know how to move between these two loves.[32]

The doctor penciled me in for surgery on February 22, the first available day after he returned from a vacation to Hawaii.

12

The Lady with the Ash-Blonde Wig

*At times I feel myself overcome by an immense tenderness for
these people around me who live in the same century.*[33]
—Albert Camus, *Notebooks 1951–1959*

Even before I had my surgery, everyone I knew urged, "Get a second
opinion." The Revlon/UCLA Breast Center was a phrase that came
up frequently in these discussions. UCLA is a dauntingly gargantuan
campus. Free street parking, a particular passion of mine, is practically
nonexistent there, and the whole notion of a public institution backed
by endowments, corporate sponsorship, and apparently a cosmetics
conglomerate—*Revlon?*—made my down-home, small-town-girl
heart quail.

I'd never even wanted a *first* opinion, but dutifully I made the
necessary requests for authorizations, frenetic phone calls, and insurance maneuvers and got myself an appointment at the Revlon/UCLA
Breast Center anyway.

Several different friends offered to go with me, but I had no desire
for company. We all have our way of moving through the world; mine
is to receive, to absorb. I can't do that and interact with another human
being at the same time. Besides, a second opinion clinic would automatically feature other people. The afternoon would be an adventure
no matter which way you cut it.

The UCLA Medical Plaza—all polished steel, glass, blond wood, and noise-absorbing carpeting—was clearly backed by some deep-pocket benefactors. The Revlon Breast Center was but one part. Once inside, I saw a youngish, shrunken guy in a wheelchair being pushed by a woman who was probably his wife, and I remembered with a start that men get cancer, too. Then I saw a sign for Pediatrics and thought, *Come ON*. Not that I hadn't known children get cancer, but the electric stab of fear I'd felt every waking and sleeping hour since the diagnosis—never mind actual physical suffering—seemed way too much for even the strongest adult, much less a small child, to bear.

I found the clinic down a couple flights of stairs. I cringingly ventured in and saw twenty or thirty women of various ages, income levels, and states of emotional balance draped over padded chairs. Presiding over the desk was a perfectly groomed young gal who looked poised to sit me down, instruct me to close my eyes, and start applying different shades of eye shadow. Instead, as was true of everyone in the medical field, her manner of greeting was to thrust into my hand a ballpoint pen and a clipboard with an impossibly thick sheaf of forms.

Settling down to fill them out gave me the same feeling I used to get in grade school before a spelling bee: namely, *I am so going to ace this*. I often simply draw a series of vertical lines through the "No" boxes on such forms: No diabetes, no heart trouble, no high blood pressure, no asthma. No, I don't smoke. No, I don't drink. It's not exactly arrogance I feel; it's more that I don't want to be a bother, and I also want to get good marks.

So when I handed in my clipboard, I was surprised to see Perky Cosmetologist Woman bearing down on me soon after. "You don't have *any* diseases?" she asked coquettishly. "I have cancer," I said flatly, not even trying to hide a small eye roll. "That's why I'm here. I assumed the question referred to diseases *other* than the cancer for which I'm seeking a second opinion."

"I saw that," a voice snickered, and I looked to my left to see a stunning blonde woman dressed to the nines Southern California style—black leather, huge ring. She might have weighed 110 pounds soaking wet, and she was tearing into a Whopper.

O.C. mall rat, I pegged her—as it turned out correctly.

"Me and my better half drove up from Newport Beach this morning," she reported, gesturing to the guy beside her, the only man in the room, a banker type in an Armani suit. "This your first time?"

I gulped. "My *only* time," I replied firmly. "I hope."

"My third, kiddo," she offered, taking a draw off a can of Diet Dr Pepper. "Yup, places like this are my home away from home." And then I saw that her shoulder-length hair was way too inert to be real: she was wearing an ash-blonde wig.

"Stare away." She laughed, and a cloud of Calvin Klein Eternity wafted over our chairs. "Double mastectomy, chemo, radiation. Bone marrow transplant, three weeks in quarantine, more chemo, every pill ever invented. That's been my life for the last ten years. Thank God for my two boys."

Her eyes misted for a second. "Troopers, those kids. Eighteen and twenty." She tore open a packet of ketchup with her teeth. "They tease the hell outta me. And they adore me."

"But . . ." I faltered and offered an unspoken prayer: *Please don't tell me you're going to die.*

A pulse beat visibly at her temple. She was so small, in her high-heeled boots, one jauntily crossed leg jittering. "At this point they can't do jack for me," she continued cheerfully. "Damn stuff's moved to my liver. We're just hoping they have some supplemental drugs that might give me a few more months. Hey, Ray, hand me my purse, willya?"

Ray handed over a quilted Chanel bag the size of a small refrigerator from which she produced a gold compact, checked her teeth, and ran a tube of hot-pink Lancôme over her lips.

I wondered how the doctors treated someone who was terminal—probably with the same impersonal, scientific coldness they treated everyone else. The system wasn't made for humans. The system was based on fear and designed for profit. Mother Teresa on the streets of Calcutta had found the only truly sane way to practice medicine (or anything else): outside all "worldly" systems. It's not that I wasn't grateful for modern medicine. It was just that by rights the whole world should have been gathered around this woman embracing her, consoling her, marveling at her, bringing her little snacks and cups of hot tea—and prayers.

Instead, she was soldiering on with the others.

"Ray baby, couldja run to the car and get my glasses. I must have left 'em on the console." Ray obediently trotted off, and she crushed her Whopper wrapper and stuffed it into the Dr Pepper can.

"Ray's a good egg," she said. "We've been together since high school. Not the brightest bulb in the box, but he makes scads of money which, trust, me, comes in handy. Not just for the medical bills but shopping does kill the pain, at least for a while."

She must have seen the stricken look on my face. "You'll be fine, kiddo," she said, leaning over to give my hand a friendly squeeze. "The fear of the unknown is the worst. Whatever happens, once you get there, it's somehow all right."

I excused myself to hit the ladies' room. When I returned, she was gone.

All afternoon I sat in strange rooms while cool hands probed my breast and murmured medical lingo. All afternoon I thought of the women who had sat staring at these same walls and heard "Stage 4" and "Nothing more we can do" and "hospice."

At the end, the "team" called me in and confirmed the diagnosis: Stage 1, Grade 1. Chance of recurrence: nine percent. Cancer was cancer, but those were pretty good odds. They didn't use the word "lucky" but I felt it, to my core.

I got dressed, said thank-yous all around, and in the hallway waited for the elevator.

The doors opened, and out stepped the lady with the ash-blonde wig, Ray trailing.

"Howdja make out, sweetie?" she called as I stepped on. "Everything all right?"

"Yeah," I said, drinking in the sight of her. "Everything's pretty much all right."

"Toldja you'd be fine," she said, beaming tenderly as the doors closed. "That's just grand."

How can you describe such heart, such class? This woman who had been through hell, who was dying—hoping someone *else* would make it.

I thought of her all the way home.

I think of her still, this woman in Prada pants who ate junk food, who liked to shop, who could have spoken a little more highly of her husband.

And each time I remember how, when Christ walked among his disciples after the Resurrection—nobody had recognized him.

13

The Anointing of the Sick

Art never responds to the wish to make it democratic; it is only for those who are willing to undergo the effort needed to understand it.[34]

—Flannery O'Connor

For Valentine's Day Tim gave me a very smart bottle of Chanel No. 5, and Judy, my friend from Hancock Park, gave me a postcard of St. Peregrine—patron saint of cancer patients—that she'd purchased at the San Juan Capistrano Mission: a photo, on a pale yellow background, of a porcelain statue of St. Peregrine wearing a floor-length black cloak. One hand pointed heavenward; the other held up a length of garment to reveal one snow white leg with a bandaged shin, and he was unmistakably, inexplicably, sticking out his tongue.

"I wonder what that's about," Judy said.

"Huh," I replied. "He's probably trying not to scream in pain."

People respond in various ways when they learn you have cancer. At the Virgin Megastore, one woman I hadn't seen in months stopped dead in her tracks, held out both arms as if she were Al Jolson about to break into "Mammy," and demanded, "Hugs! HUGS!" A loud redhead named Yosemite approached me one morning in Ralphs Grocery and ordered in a throaty voice, "Get in a support group and keep going even when your treatment's over. Eighteen years later I still go—even though everyone from the original group has died but me."

And one night not long after being diagnosed, I received a call from my friend Cedric. Cedric said he was sorry about my cancer, then proceeded to inform me that though the fact was by no means generally known, most people were saturated with a sense of guilt and self-loathing so intense that they not only brought serious illnesses upon themselves but also ended up dying of them because they didn't think they deserved to get well. We had no idea of the power of healing we could unleash by ridding ourselves of this guilt, he said.

So far, so good—sort of—but then he got all somber and wizardy, hinting at the secrets of the universe and offering to let me in on an incredibly powerful method of prayer that I had to be sworn to secrecy not to tell anyone about because in the wrong hands a tremendous amount of damage could be done. This prayer had been used by many people I knew (*Like who?* I wondered. *Why hadn't they told me about it?*), including a friend of his who would never lie to him and used it to miraculously cure himself of terminal cancer. But the thing about this prayer was that it would work only if you truly wanted to live. Another friend had tried the prayer and failed: he had died because he couldn't bring himself to confront the fact that he didn't truly want to live.

"Can you honestly tell me, Heather," Cedric whispered, "right now, this minute, do you even know, are you even aware enough, to say whether you TRULY WANT TO LIVE?"

I stifled the urge to say, "*No, but I truly want you to shut up.*" The tone of the conversation had turned so creepy I'd started making the sign of the cross over myself, as if warding off a hex. I was no expert, but could the fruits of any real prayer lead you to call a person with cancer and inform him that the fault was his? Could the fruits of any real prayer lead you to ambush a carcinoma-ridden friend with the news that her existential ambivalence was going to kill her? Wouldn't the fruits of real prayer lead you to see that the most compassionate thing you could do for a sick person would be to say that you were dreadfully sorry, then leave the person to find his or her own way?

I'm usually hyperanxious to avoid "hurting people's feelings," but I'd reached my limit. "Listen, Cedric," I finally said, "I know you're only trying to help, and I appreciate your calling, but you're being preachy and patronizing and you're making me very, very nervous."

I think I might have felt several cancer cells dying even as the words issued from my mouth. And then—I hung up.

One name I couldn't seem to avoid in the Cancer Universe was Bernie Siegel, a doctor interested in the mind-body approach to illness who had written, among other things, a bestseller called *Peace, Love, and Healing.*

I paid a buck at a used-book store for a copy and read the whole thing through the next morning. I'd had moderately high hopes, but the stories were so pat and life-affirming that I had a hard time believing they were real. The pop psychology questionnaires were strictly for the astrology set—"Do you want to live to be a hundred?"[35] for example, or "Why do you need your illness, and what benefits do you derive from it?"[36] And the way Bernie envisioned leading people to "Super Health" seemed significantly less than natural: "At the vanguard of this new science are the researchers who are studying a group of peptides known as growth factors, which are naturally occurring substances in our bodies now being cloned through the techniques of genetic engineering."[37]

The book was full of hopelessly broad generalizations that were not even true; for example, "People who have cancer . . . tend to be people who have always put other people first. They need to be liked."[38] (People without cancer don't need to be liked? Selfish jerks never get cancer?) Bernie cited with approval some of the patients who had finally started putting themselves first: the woman with breast cancer who had bought herself a thoroughbred horse ("A present I have waited for every Christmas since childhood. I finally got it!");[39] the gal who, since being given a death sentence, had "traveled widely," "visited thirty or more museums," gone away for "weekends of dancing, swimming, flirting, etc." and "most important," had found "a wonderful boyfriend who takes me out to dinner and the movies and with whom I have a fulfilling sex life."[40]

This penchant for quick-and-easy answers (which I soon learned characterized 95 percent of the "healing" literature) aroused my deepest suspicions. I had certainly done my share of being a people-pleasing doormat, but there was not a doubt in my mind that at the end of my life, I was going to regret not failing to think enough about myself but failing to think enough about others. Nobody begrudges a dying person a longed-for thoroughbred, but wouldn't the truly transformative event be to bestow the nag upon, say, some poor leukemic kid who looked as if she were going to have even less of a chance than you? Wouldn't the more sublime conversion consist not in the cultivation of a "fulfilling" sex life but, as it had for St. Francis of Assisi, in embracing a leper? Wouldn't the legacy you wanted to contemplate from your deathbed be not so much having visited thirty or more museums but having visited some pariah of a prisoner or an inmate in a psych ward or your brother who your mother had always liked best and whom you knew would never in a million years conceive of visiting you?

I wholly supported self-care, but I was also always reaching for what, if anything, lay beyond self-care. "What is born of the flesh is flesh, and what is born of the Spirit is spirit. . . . The wind blows where it chooses, and you hear the sound of it, but you do not know where it comes from or where it goes. So it is with everyone who is born of the Spirit" (John 3:6, 8).

The only "rebirth" I had ever experienced had come after years of painful and frustrating self-examination, a concerted effort to alter my thinking and behavior, and an entirely unmerited influx of grace. Bernie's patients, by contrast, had dealt with their life-threatening illnesses by smiling ruefully, squaring their shoulders, and changing overnight into models of cooperation, calm, and charity.

A fellow named Kevin, for instance, had died in his thirties of a rare genetic disease. First, however, he had attended Bernie's support groups, done visualization exercises that had been specially tailored by Bernie to the needs of his disease, and watched Bernie's videotapes on healing. As a consequence, Kevin had become "positive," "helpful," and "accepting," with a "beautiful smile" for everyone.[41] Kevin had joined up. Kevin had transformed himself into Bernie's vision of mental health. Kevin had become part of Bernie's "exceptional patient" program.

Aside from the incongruity between so-called spirituality on the one hand and shilling for money on the other, why—in addition to the appalling burden of, say, being in unspeakable pain and at the very least knowing you possibly stood to die soon—did you have to be an exceptional patient? Why not be just an ordinary patient, a mediocre patient, a bewildered, pissed-off patient?

Kevin's sister had died of the same rare genetic disease Kevin had but—without the benefit of any of Bernie's products—bitter and withdrawn from first to last. Bernie, of course, thoroughly disapproved: "The way she died, with such anger, made it hard on all members of her extended family, on her caregivers, and on herself."[42] But my own thought was that here at last was someone with whom I could thoroughly relate. If I were on my deathbed and some glad-handing, hokey-bestseller-writing doctor were urging me to join his "exceptional patient" support group, I would have been bitter and withdrawn too.

There's nothing wrong with being cheerful, and my hat was off to anyone who had found solace in *Peace, Love, and Healing*. But I'd cast my lot with the sister who raged against the dying of the light rather than with Kevin, the perfect brother who dutifully bought all of Bernie Siegel's books.

More to the point, I'd cast my lot with Christ, which was why, a couple of days before surgery, I went up to St. Basil's for a visit with my beloved Father Terry. Father Terry is tall and thin, and this particular day was nicely turned out in a pressed Ralph Lauren shirt and dark green slacks.

The rectory, on the other hand, appeared to have been untouched since around 1962 (which I actually kind of liked) and featured over-sized lamps with nubby beige shades, overtinted photos of past resident priests, and kidney-shaped ashtrays of orange plastic.

"So what's up?" he asked, tilting in his Naugahyde recliner.

"Fear, what else?" I said, and proceeded to describe a few of them: dying on the operating table, living only to die a painful death later. I also hadn't realized that good health and a relatively unblemished body were so much a part of my identity.

"Illness causes a fundamental change in identity," Father Terry pointed out, "just as stopping drinking does, so of course that feels scary."

He wasn't about to come out next and say, "Join the club, you're not the only sick person in the world" or "You can be of service even when you're dying" or "You wouldn't believe the joy and faith with which

I've seen people walk through illnesses ten times worse than what it looks like you've got."

Instead, he told a couple of stories. He told about how he had recently visited an eleven-year-old girl with leukemia and that it had been difficult to know what to say because he figured she probably knew way more about life at that point than he did. He told about a friend of his, an advertising executive who'd been at St. John's Health Center over in Santa Monica for a couple of years before dying of cancer. Once, when Terry was visiting, the guy had started talking, then trailed off and said, "I can't remember the ends of things anymore. I can barely even pray. I just look over there"—he pointed to the crucifix that was hanging on the wall—"and sort of throw the names of my friends at it."

As long as even one person in the world were praying like that, I figured, we were saved. Unlike the power-of-positive-thinking kind of prayer, the fruit of real prayer did not depend on whether you lived or died. The fruit of real prayer was self-surrender, abandonment, a voluntary climbing up on the pyre to be consumed by the blaze of God's mercy. Not that I was anywhere near that point myself; this guy had been on his deathbed praying for his friends, and I was worried because I might not get to play tennis and gaze at my beautiful hardwood floors for the next fifty years.

Just when I was starting to feel like a big, self-pitying baby who should have been thanking my lucky stars for even being able to breathe, Father Terry asked, "Would you like to receive the Anointing of the Sick?"

The Anointing of the Sick is one of the seven sacraments of the Catholic Church, and I'd consulted my *Catechism* the week before to ascertain whether I qualified.

> By the sacred anointing of the sick and the prayer of the priests
> the whole Church commends those who are ill to the suffering

and glorified Lord, that he may raise them up and save them [Section 1499]. . . . She believes in the life-giving presence of Christ, the physician of souls and bodies [Section 1509]. . . . It is fitting to receive the Anointing of the Sick just prior to a serious operation' [Section 1515].

I'd figured that a lumpectomy probably didn't qualify as serious, but as Father Terry pointed out, "What you have is life-threatening with a small *t*." Because I had wanted the sacrament but had been afraid that asking would be an imposition, the offer was a deep and unexpected blessing.

"I would love that more than anything," I told him. "It may be a smallish surgery, but it's the first surgery I've ever had."

So he went out to the parking lot, where his Honda was parked, and brought in a flat black leather case the size of a Bible. A faraway look came into his eyes, as he no doubt pictured countless long-ago visits to the sick, the bedridden, the dying. "I've been carrying this around for thirty-five years," he said.

"Really? What's in it?" I asked nosily, and he unzipped around the edge and showed me the ivory silk lining, the worn grosgrain ribbons, the frilled pockets holding a gold pyx for the Blessed Sacrament, a tiny blue enameled box for holy oil, and a plastic container filled with cotton balls.

Then he put a purple stole around his shoulders, opened a dog-eared green book called *Pastoral Care of the Sick*, and began:

"The peace of the Lord be with you always."

"And also with you."

Together, we prayed the Penitential Rite:

"I confess to almighty God, and to you, my brothers and sisters . . ."

He laid his hands on my head and said:

"At sunset, all who had people sick with various diseases brought them to him. He laid his hands on each of them and cured them" (Luke 4:40).

Then he made the Sign of the Cross in oil on my forehead:

"Through this holy anointing may the Lord in his love and mercy help you with the grace of the Holy Spirit."

"Amen."

He anointed my palms, first the right, then the left, also with the Sign of the Cross:

"May the Lord who frees you from sin save you and raise you up."

"Amen."

The oil warm on my palms, I reflected that anointing, unlike Cedric's prayer, was not only for the spiritually elite, and unlike Bernie Siegel's "exceptional patient" program, was not a marketing device. Unlike the cutting, burning, and poisoning the medical profession had to offer, the Church offered a gentle anointing with holy oil, the curative truth of the Gospels, prayers for grace. Unlike the property-, power-, and prestige-based culture, Christ found and addressed your deepest soul.

I did not believe the Anointing would protect me from harm or death, or confer some special status, or give rise to some miracle of physical healing. I believed that the Anointing consecrated my illness to the larger community. I believed the Anointing acknowledged that sickness is, at its deepest level, a mystical phenomenon. I believed that if I were to die of my illness, the Anointing would be the first step in offering my death to the world.

14

Under the Knife

It's no real pleasure in life.[43]
—The Misfit, from the Flannery O'Connor short story
"A Good Man Is Hard to Find"

The morning of my surgery, Tim and I started for the hospital at six-thirty, the familiar sights—the day laborers hanging out at San Marino and Ardmore, the crack hotels around Bonnie Brae as we approached downtown—seeming even more grubbily human and precious than usual because, though I hoped to be going home that afternoon, one never knew. If the crackheads and drunks were to be the last people among whom I walked, they were my people, more or less, and God bless us all. Tim and I found a very nice free space to park in front of a sagging building on whose front stoop several early risers were smoking a joint and swilling Tecate, and walked the few blocks to the hospital.

Thrilled that the weeks-long anticipatory dread was finally nearing an end, I felt almost jaunty. The admitting desk was manned by an African-American male who was built like a refrigerator. "How do," I announced brightly. "I'm going under the knife today!"

I'd imagined being left to molder in a back hallway, but to my utter gratification and surprise, I was instead whisked through pre-op with dispatch, courtesy, even concern. After I was admitted and had my blood drawn, a pleasant orderly named Lizardo took me upstairs for a couple of mammograms and a chest X-ray (where I spotted the familiar mammogram tech) and led me to ultrasound, where a large group crowded around my poor, unsuspecting breast.

These included a Dr. Park, who appeared to be approximately twelve years of age; a Dr. Dianne Ditka, who looked like an anorectic B-movie actress; and several hangers-on who introduced themselves by first name only. This eager team took turns running a gel-coated cable over the area above my tumor and jostling for a look at the monitor: "Can you see it? No, left, left! Three o'clock, see it, right there!" While I suppressed the urge to ask Dr. Park if he'd yet started shaving, he sprayed on some Lidocaine and proceeded to insert a thin wire—a marker for the surgery—and he cheerfully informed me that I was then expected to walk around for the next several hours with this wire hanging out of my breast.

In this state, I was escorted to an examining table for some real torture: four injections of radium dye into what felt like the deepest core of my breast, an ordeal so painful that on the fourth stab, tears spontaneously leaked forth from beneath my clamped-shut eyelids. Dr. Ditka—who had long bleached-blonde hair, a face so white it appeared to have been powdered with cornstarch, and apparently the only heart in the room—comfortingly rubbed my shoulder and said everything would be all right, and after a while, everything was.

Next I was placed on a gurney and rolled over to nuclear medicine, where for two interminable hours I lay motionless while a tech trained the giant eye of a metal machine at various points on my breast. A companionable Doctor Rasheesh, who wore shirtsleeves and a comb-over, came around every so often and in a low-key, calming voice delivered a thumbnail description of nuclear medicine (something to do with isotopes: the injected radioactive dye went to various parts of your body, enabling them to pinpoint, among other things, cancer sites);

explained what he was doing (watching the dye move through my bloodstream); and remarked that cracking the cancer code must surely only be a matter of time, but he wished to hell the time would come sooner. "Cancer is just one of those little bumps on the road of life," he mused.

A philosophizing doctor! I liked that (though easy for him to say), especially as my stint as a lawyer had not instilled confidence in any profession: not business, not education, not medicine, and most definitely not the law. I kept thinking about a medical malpractice case I'd once worked on, in which the plaintiff was the widow of a strapping man who'd gone in for routine, outpatient foot surgery and, while she'd waited for him to emerge so they could go to lunch, had died on the table.

At one point Ricketts himself made an appearance, dressed to the nines in street clothes and as full of tactless asides as ever. Grasping the wire protruding from my breast, he did a double take and leered, "Better you than me," but I was glad to see him all the same and touched, even if the gesture was only a professional courtesy, that he'd made the effort. Dr. Rasheesh's assistant was a lovely large gal with a lilting Caribbean accent who smelled of soap and spearmint and was a pleasure in every way. Nonetheless, by eleven o'clock I had such excruciating pains shooting down my lower back from being immobilized for so long that I was dying to go get carved up, just for a change of pace.

Being wheeled up to surgery got me not only out of nuclear medicine but also reunited with Tim, who'd been faithfully standing by. They parked the two of us in a small curtained-off area and, as I began to undress, a nurse in green scrubs appeared, rubbed her hands together like a praying mantis scraping its front legs, and announced, "We've been waiting for you!"

She instructed me to take off everything, including my jewelry and panties. As I handed over my watch and thirty-five-dollar gold wedding band to Tim, I whispered, "Why panties? They're going to molest me, I know it."

The nurse thrust an IV line into the back of my hand and the anesthesiologist came by to ask if I wore dentures or contact lenses, to which I answered no on both counts. "Be right back," he said, adjusting his fabric shower cap. "We're almost ready."

I turned to Tim. Notoriously overwrought at hellos and especially at good-byes, I realized that the kind thing might be for once not to act like Bette Davis in the final scene of *Now, Voyager.* "If anything happens, honey, I love you with all my heart," I told him. "And get married again right away. You need serious taking care of."

"I love you, too," he said. "And if you don't come out, it will be really, really great, I mean it will be really sad, when I get all your money." (The nest egg I'd saved from lawyering, which supported my writing and I guarded like a hawk, was a standing joke between us. On the day of a friend's lumpectomy, her husband had arranged with the surgeon to sneak into the operating room and slip a diamond bracelet on her wrist. Mine, I reflected, would probably steal my wallet).

All the same, I knew he was nervous: his hands were clammy when he took mine, and Tim never had clammy hands. He was still holding them when the anesthesiologist came back and told me to lie down on the gurney.

"This will just take the edge off," the guy said, popping something into the IV line, and as I waved good-bye to Tim, he wheeled me into a room where Barbra Streisand was singing and a man in a pale blue mask sat staring from a stool, and the ceiling was covered with huge bright rectangular lights, and I began praying the ancient lines known in the Church as the Animi Christi:

> Soul of Christ, sanctify me.
> Body of Christ, save me.
> Blood of Christ, inebriate me.

Water from the side of Christ, wash me.
Passion of Christ, strengthen me.
O good Jesus, hear me.
Within Thy wounds, hide me. . .

Next thing I knew, I was in the recovery room asking, "Can I go home? Are they going to let me go home?" Because even out cold, the whole time I'd been lost in the ether, through my addled brain had run a single refrain—If they let me go home, that means they only had to take out one node; that means my nodes were clean—and some angel nurse said, "Yes, they're going to let you go home," and I started crying.

"What's the matter?" she asked, and I couldn't really explain so I said, "A lot of emotion," and left it at that. I flexed my hand under the blanket to find that, miraculously, the nerves were still connected, that I wasn't crippled, and when I looked up again, Staggers was there. I gazed lovingly upon his impassive face, grabbed his hand with my sweaty paw and croaked, "All clear? Everything came out all right?" He nodded and the next second, seemingly, was gone.

The beds around me, I was now sentient enough to notice, were filled with other poor souls who had also been cut up and were just coming around, mostly old people who in no way, shape, or form should have had to undergo anything as grim and painful as surgery. I myself was totally nauseated, and there is really nothing worse than nausea, no possible way to get comfortable or formulate any other thought than a nausea thought. Home—four miles away—seemed like the other side of the universe, impossibly beyond reach.

After a while Tim appeared, and the angel nurse helped me up. Getting dressed took forever: I tortuously inched the bad arm into the sleeve of my sweater, buttoned up wrong, left my pants unzipped. Tim went ahead to bring around the truck, and an orderly rolled up to the door of the bathroom with a wheelchair, took me down in the elevator, and helped bundle me in.

The hour was half past four as we left—where had the day gone?—with a gray sky full of scudding clouds and the wind whipping up. My head felt as fragile as an egg, and I carefully trained my gaze straight ahead as we drove down Olympic, past the neon strip malls of Shiseido outlets, saunas, billiard halls. Just as we pulled into the alley behind our apartment, I brought up the entire contents of my stomach: half a cup of bright blue, totally clear liquid that looked exactly like Windex.

"What is that?" I said. We decided it was either anesthetic or radioactive dye because this color was found in no natural foodstuff.

Tim helped me hobble upstairs, where I ate a bowl of cream of mushroom soup, half a pint of chocolate sorbet, and a Vicodin and almost immediately felt a thousand percent better. Everything seemed suddenly wondrous: the Stargazer lilies on the coffee table, the chirping of the crickets in the courtyard, food. That you could go to the store and buy a container of sorbet, bring it home, spoon it into one of the hand-painted blue-and-gold pottery bowls we'd brought home from Guadalajara seemed the most interesting and delightful thing in the world. Who cared that a chunk was gone from my breast? So what if I had cancer? I was still alive! I was breathing! "I feel so good," I kept telling Tim, "I can't believe how good I feel!"

I was starting to think I'd reached some pinnacle of spiritual growth where even pain made me grateful, but then Tim pointed out that I could probably thank the Vicodin. With my track record, this was an area about which I had to be a teensy bit careful. So I took only one more, thanking God with practically every breath, and after that I switched to Tylenol.

15

Fool for Christ

Mysticism remains the great science and the great art, the only power capable of synthesizing the riches accumulated by other forms of human activity.[44]
—Teilhard de Chardin, September 9, 1923

Christ is interesting, but he's not explicable. Christ is not a theory; Christ is an event, an invitation. As the German theologian Karl Rahner observed, "Tomorrow's devout person will either be a mystic—someone who has 'experienced' something—or they will not be devout at all."[45]

Mysticism, I'd come to see, is no vague abstraction; mysticism, to me, was simply a way of saying that the entire thrust of Christianity is love. To follow Christ makes no sense without love. The whole Way, Truth, and Life is about being in love with Christ—which is to say, being in love with reality. "This Jesus is 'the stone that was rejected by you, the builders; it has become the cornerstone'" (Acts 4:11). Exactly where I thought Christ couldn't be—the boring homily, the screaming kids, the sexual obsession, the doubt, the fear: that's where he most was.

We can't contain our love, and so, enculturated from birth, we're embarrassed by our love, we belittle our love, we hide our love. Or we let even the best-intentioned love be reduced to all kinds of things that are, or were in the beginning, oriented toward love but that become less than, or misguided forms of, love. Our desire to be good becomes perfectionism, for example; or our hunger for righteousness turns us self-righteous; or our genuine desire to spread the Gospel subtly morphs into a desire to promote ourselves.

To follow Christ, though, is no career move. The mark of authentic conversion is that it costs you something, not that it gains you something. So to try to become, say, "pro-life" or anti-war, or a Catholic convert celebrity perhaps would be something, but it would not be Christianity. I'd seen early on that to slant my work politically, to have an axe to grind, to identify myself primarily as the promoter of a movement, issue, or cause would have been to be a money changer in the temple. It would be to try to make a name for myself, to cultivate a reputation, to strive for notoriety based not on my love but on my "views."

Long ago I had seen that both the Catholic right and the Catholic left were simply variations on "the world" in which the goals were power, prestige, efficiency, triumph, and to shame or bully other people into changing without changing one iota yourself. The Catholic media that trafficked in incessant, opinion-driven, vitriolic "discussion" seemed to me to have very little, if anything, to do with Christ. Keep my own side of the street clean and pray—pray for us all—was more my idea.

The people who wore their giant aborted-fetus buttons—to take one of the more unfortunate examples of the religious right—reminded me of the Pharisees who prayed loudly on the street corners and wore their phylacteries long. "We care," they proclaim; they insist. "We care more than you do. We're more outraged than you are. We're saved and you're not."

That's why I steered clear of the religious right.

The religious left, on the other hand, was based on faux love. Artificial birth control, the abolition of priestly celibacy, sex outside marriage: all were supposedly an increase of love. Two people slept together to see whether they were compatible, thereby (supposedly) saving the world from slews of unhappy unions: that was an increase in love, the thinking went. But more and more I saw that this kind of "love" urges people to take a shortcut to avoid suffering, which is to say to miss out on coming fully awake. It's the "love" that says, "I think you're too delicate to face the highest truth and live it out. I don't think you're strong enough, or mature enough, to take in the whole picture, to hold the full tension of the suffering of the world before you; I don't trust you to recognize that to aim for anything lower than the highest is to contribute to that suffering and, as much to the point, to deprive yourself of the highest joy. So if a kid you conceive might be 'unwanted,' abort him or her. If an old person strikes you as no longer serving any 'useful purpose,' help him or her to commit suicide."

Unfortunately, the underlying idea, if you follow it through—and you don't have to follow it very far—is "Exterminate or annihilate people who are suffering or might stand to suffer." Which in the end is going to be everybody, because the human condition is suffering. Christ, nailed to a cross above the altar of every Catholic Church in the world, is simply the image of the human condition. You can't annihilate suffering; you can only share in it. You can only try to refrain from contributing to it.

Which was one reason that the teachings of the Church on sex, which once had seemed unthinking and rigid, now struck me instead as beautifully reflective of the fact that everybody—married, single, straight, gay, young, old—is invited to contribute to the human family. Everyone has a part to play in inviting, welcoming, rejoicing in, marveling at, and supporting new life and all life. Everyone can offer his or her sexuality toward the healing of the festering sexual wound at the heart of humankind.

Suffering always stems from or is exacerbated by a lack of love, and love is grounded in family and the holiness of sex and the sacrament of marriage. And thus our life's work, no matter what our station, is to welcome, support, rejoice in, marvel at, and support new life and all life: in charity, in integrity, in truth. Which requires sacrifice, on everybody's part.

So much sacrifice, in fact, that I, for one, was way too busy to get overly exercised about whether to, say, bring back the Latin Mass or to overfocus on partisan politics or to clamor for reform in the hierarchy. I tended to look at the people who were always railing against the Church (from either side) and think: How in any way is the Church impinging upon your freedom? Are the Papal police hauling you into court? Is Rome telling you anything other than at the last day you will be judged by how you treated the least of these, which includes not just the unborn or the illegal immigrant or the prisoner on death row or whoever else you've adopted as your cause, but the person on the other side of the fence: your "enemy"? If the Church started saying, you can't pray, you can't go to Confession, you're not allowed to be emotionally or sexually responsible, and you are obligated to hate your enemy, I'd start to worry.

As it was, I was always a little taken aback by the complete lack of affection, often within her own ranks, for the Church. To me, the Church was a little like having an alcoholic mother: majestic one minute and engaging in some cringingly non-Christlike behavior the next. But no matter what, she was your Mother. No matter what, you love your mother. And the way you love her is you notice when she goes wrong, you grieve for her, and then you silently resolve to help her do a little better. You don't pretend not to see her faults and get all self-righteous and militaristic if someone attacks her—but you also don't kick her when she's down.

I think the way we feel about the Church is very much an indication of how we feel, in our hearts, about the least of our brothers and sisters. "You only love God as much as you love the person you love least," activist Dorothy Day once quoted a priest friend. And by extension, my sense was that I loved God about as much as I loved His Church—and the people in it.

Like the Cross, the Church could neither be promoted nor defended. Like the Cross, she could only be loved. We followers of Christ did not come to church striving for efficiency or results, or to swagger and preen and lord it over the rest of the world. We came as sinners, as beggars. We came hungering and thirsting. We came: the blind, the deaf, the halt, the leprous, the demoniacs, the desperate, the lost, the lonely. We did not have our political views to offer; we had Christ. We did not have convincing arguments; we had our wounds, our holy longing, our groping in the dark. We didn't have clever op-eds; we had our bodies, our puny desire to be good, our lurching, guaranteed-to-fall-short striving for purity.

Here's how I knew I was very, very slowly becoming a follower of Christ. I was willing to be seen less, not more. I began to want to be quieter, not louder. I found myself making tiny sacrifices: fasting from meat for a day or giving the three bucks I would have spent at Starbucks to a homeless person. I found myself experiencing tiny moments of joy. I found myself mysteriously, ever more deeply drawn to Confession, to Mass. More and more I asked different questions from those the world asked. I looked for a different kind of result. I served a different master.

Or as Cardinal Emmanuel Célistin Suhard, Archbishop of Paris from 1940–1949, observed: "To be a witness does not consist in engaging in propaganda or even in stirring people up, but in being a living mystery; it means to live in such a way that one's life would not make sense if God did not exist."[46]

16

St. Andrew's Abbey

*To lead a truly spiritual life while remaining in perfect health
physically and psychically—this no man can do.*[47]
—Franz Kafka

The morning after my surgery, the nurse from the recovery room
called to see how I was feeling, a touch I deeply appreciated. Afterward, Tim sat me in a warm tub and washed my tummy and arms,
then had me kneel while he did my hair. What am I learning from
this? I thought. Not to be so anxious? That way less is expected of me
than I think?

Monday, as I hovered by the phone, Staggers called and uttered the
miraculous words: my nodes were definitely clear. There was a patronizing note about him, a strain around the edges of his professional
calm—the way he answered my questions with an unspoken tone of
"If you would just shut up and listen to me, the omniscient expert,
I will tell you all that you, an ignorant, hysterical laywoman, need
to know or are capable of absorbing"—but what could I do? I could
hardly expect him to have experienced the terror and angst of breast
cancer.

For my part, I had already done enough research to be frothing at
the mouth at the prospect of learning my estrogen and progesterone
receptor status and my HER2/neu and S-phase status—the "markers"

used to predict whether and how fast the cancer was likely to spread—and I could hardly wait to hear his treatment recommendations.

That, of course, all had to be done in person: I took the first available appointment for the following week.

Learning that my lymph nodes were clear was a major, major relief, but I still had invasive breast cancer; I still didn't have the full pathology report, and depending upon which set of statistics were to be believed, up to 55 percent of all breast-cancer patients still died within ten years of being diagnosed.

I needed some time alone in which to digest the events of the past month. St. Andrew's Abbey, the Benedictine monastery where I'd had a previous retreat scheduled and cancelled, was usually booked weeks in advance, but on the spur of the moment I called and lucked out. They had a room available for three nights, starting the following day.

So the next afternoon I drove a couple of hours northeast of the city, through the Angeles Forest to the Pearblossom Highway and on through the western Mojave to the tiny desert town of Valyermo. The abbey, located in a seven-hundred-acre valley of Lombardy poplars, apple trees, and hiking trails, comprised several modest buildings: the monks' quarters, two dormitories of spartan but comfortable rooms, a large common area and dining hall, and the nerve center—the chapel.

Upon arriving, I looked around my room—concrete floor, cinder-block walls, a small wooden crucifix—and thought, *Ah . . . home. . . .* On the desk was a laminated schedule reading, "The Horarium or daily schedule at Valyermo is a modern adaptation of the cycle of prayer and work prescribed by St. Benedict in his Rule. Periods of common and private prayer, manual labor and study are intertwined, so that the entire day can take on the character of Divine Presence."

The first night I went to bed early. At six the next morning I joined the monks in chapel, then hiked for an hour, watching the morning light make halos around the spines of cholla cacti and glow pink through the ears of baby rabbits. The air was chilly—Valyermo is "high" desert—and back in my room after breakfast, I pulled a rocking chair up to the flame of the gas heater and prepared to do some hard thinking.

So far all my energy had gone to assimilating the fact that I had cancer at all. Now that I had room to breathe, the questions that had been roiling beneath the surface for weeks broke through: Why? How? What, if anything, did having cancer mean?

I'd brought a pile of articles and books, but from my research, I already knew the basic cancer-causation theories. There was the genetic theory, but that didn't seem to apply to me. My older cousin Patty had been diagnosed the year before, but none of my first-degree relatives (sisters, mother) ever had, and cancer of any kind didn't seem to run in the family (though as my younger sister remarked, apropos of the pathologically secretive streak that ran through both sides of our bloodline, "How would we know?"). There was the toxic universe theory, which held that the food we eat, the water we drink, and the air we breathe were all so loaded with poison we might as well just give up and get measured for a coffin. As a resident of L.A., this struck me as a definite possibility. Still, the question remained, If the whole world was toxic, why had I gotten it? Why hadn't everybody?

No, what I really had to come to grips with was the hideous fact, emblazoned across every piece of research I'd read to date, that heavy drinking, birth-control pills, and abortions had all been linked to breast cancer—that I may, in other words, have at least partly contributed to the situation myself. I may not have, too; my cancer may just have been the bad luck of the draw, but either way, examining my conscience, sexual/emotional history, and interpersonal relationships could only help. At all costs I wanted to avoid the idea of cancer as payback from a vengeful, malevolent God, so I decided to sit down at the desk and, with a small wooden crucifix on the cinder-block wall above me, try to work out my thoughts on paper.

In spite of my matter-of-fact approach to "personal care," even I had come to subscribe over the years to some kind of mind-body connection; had come to see, for example, that the backaches and insomnia that sometimes plagued me were no doubt triggered by anxiety. I will also say that it's very difficult, when you have cancer, not to ask, Is it my fault? Did I somehow bring this on myself? Those were the questions my pen formed first, and though I basically knew better, what emerged as I wrote were the first stirrings of the idea that cancer, like alcoholism—like any physical illness—has an emotional and spiritual dimension.

The scientific explanation for why taking birth-control pills and having abortions may have figured into the equation was that breast cancer seemed to be connected—nobody was exactly sure why or how—with increased estrogen levels. But maybe the ultimate underlying or, at the very least, connected, reason was that all those years of emotional anguish (the tumor had, after all, been found next to my heart), those years of treating myself and other people like objects, had been bound to eventually manifest somehow. Maybe you can't violate someone else's body without the violence redounding to your own. Maybe my intuition, back in my twenties, that if I ever got sick the illness would implicate my reproductive system, had arisen from the fact that even then I knew that my deepest, most secret psychic wounds were going to be sexual.

One of my worst wounds was the huge wound I had inflicted on my marriage by aborting the child I'd conceived with Tim. I had never come out and admitted it, even to myself, that the abortion (my third) I'd had ten years ago, just before we'd been married had inflicted a terrible, terrible wound on us. The decision had been mine—I'd been newly sober; we were broke—and though Tim had concurred, I saw now that on some level all along I had blamed him. I had never fully forgiven him for being just as scared and overwhelmed as me and for having just as closed a heart. That doctors—purportedly bound by the Hippocratic oath to "do no harm"—had performed my abortions, it occurred to me now, also may have contributed to my tendency to view the medical profession with less than unalloyed trust. Not that I blamed the doctors, but in fact, one line of the original oath runs: "I will not give a lethal drug to anyone if I am asked, nor will I advise such a plan; and similarly I will not give a woman a pessary to cause an abortion."[48]

The decision to abort had sprung from my fear that I was neither worthy of love nor capable of love (and that there wouldn't be enough money), and the abortion, of course, had only exacerbated the fear. What made matters worse was that as the years passed, I saw what an incredible father Tim would have been, that he would have loved having children. And instead of having compassion for him, I had been hard on both of us. Just recently I'd been thinking that at this stage of my life, I might finally have been able to welcome a child. That probably would be one of the regrets of my life: that I'd never had children (though I also suspected I may have subconsciously chosen being a writer over being a mother, knowing that I would have been incapable of doing both). But even to have reached the point where I could see how amazing having a child might have been represented some form of progress. To see that my perspective had been skewed, that I'd blamed Tim for my own shortcomings, was at least a small step toward metanoia: the opening of the heart, to counter the heart that closes around guilt, sin, hurt.

Outside my window, the coin-like leaves of an aspen trembled in the breeze. I'd confessed my abortions when I'd come into the Church, but even the Sacrament of Reconciliation couldn't make me feel forgiven. I'd recently learned that *reconcile*, from the root word *cilia*, means to come eyelash to eyelash again with another. I'd reconciled myself in some sense to God, but I wondered now if sorrow, shame, and guilt had prevented me all these years from coming eyelash to eyelash with myself.

I sat, lost in thought, and then—I'm not sure what possessed me—I went into the bathroom, stood in front of the medicine cabinet for about ten minutes, and just looked at my face. I'm not sure that in my whole life I had ever once looked at myself in the mirror without instinctively putting on the mask we wear for others, and maybe even more for ourselves. First, horror: I looked so old. There were caverns on either side of my mouth; my hair was whacked.

Nothing happened. I didn't see my inner beauty; I didn't feel any huge rush of love for myself. But I kept staring, and after a while I was able to look into my own eyes and smile a kind of cockeyed, wanly welcoming smile. It was a start.

Mass at St. Andrew's, celebrated at noon that day, seemed an especially holy event: the monks slowly processing into the chapel in their ivory robes, the sun illuminating the tangerine and pale purple hunks of stained glass, the Eucharist dispensed with the unhurried reverence and hushed solemnity it deserved.

Taking the Host into my cupped hands, watching the monks dish out soup in the dining hall afterward, sitting by my window as the afternoon shadows lengthened—and the tape beneath my shirt pulling at the gauze I hadn't yet dared lift—I thought of the Body broken in exchange for our own brokenness: our mistakes, our lack of faith, our fear.

Lying in bed that night, pondering further the possible spiritual dimension of illness, I realized that most of the writers I admired had suffered from and/or died of debilitating diseases: TB, lupus, alcoholism.

Franz Kafka, for one, had been convinced that illness was only the physical manifestation of a much deeper, psychic conflict. Shortly after being diagnosed with tuberculosis, he had written to a friend, "I am constantly seeking an explanation for this disease, for I did not seek it. Sometimes it seems to me that my brain and lungs came to an agreement without my knowledge. 'Things can't go on this way,' said the brain, and after five years the lungs said they were ready to help."[49]

Kafka had always been a particular hero of mine. No one hovered with quite such excruciating tension on the edge of despair; no one subjected his characters quite so pitilessly to the unrelenting exile of the human condition; no one imparted such a tremulous sense of life as a God-haunted, waking-sleeping nightmare.

After "The Metamorphosis"—before which, of course, the world must simply bow its head—to me his most gripping story was "In the Penal Colony." The four allegorical characters—the traveler, the officer, the condemned, and the soldier—are gathered around an instrument of torture, now poised for its last run: a frightful device consisting of a bed to which the condemned is strapped while the Harrow, two sets of quivering, specially configured needles, "spell out" on his body the words of the disobeyed law.

The officer is proud to have overseen many such executions. Already nostalgic for the days when all prisoners were judged automatically guilty, with no trial, he waxes poetic about the way, just before death, the exhausted faces of even the most dull-witted convicts are transformed as they "absorb" the Harrow's ghastly, individually designed message. Coveting a similar religious experience for himself, he pardons the condemned, configures the harrow to spell out "BE JUST," and straps himself in. Due to its advanced state of disrepair, however, the machine malfunctions and brutally, gruesomely stabs him to death. (Love Franz!)

I had always thought of the Harrow as a symbol of life as undeserved, dumbly endured torture—of being on trial for an offense we don't remember committing, of being punished for simply existing. But from my bed at St. Andrew's that night, I saw that it could more specifically be a metaphor for the way we bear on our bodies the ravages of our psycho-spiritual shortcomings—even, or perhaps especially, the ones so deeply ingrained, so patently not "our fault," that they seem incapable of correction: the tumors on the lungs of a smoker who craves nicotine to quiet nerves set raw by childhood beatings; the steel pins in the shoulder of a motorcyclist who, called "Faggot" as a teenager, takes up drag racing to prove his manliness; the gangrene on the legs of my diabetic father, who had ignored the ulcerated sores on his feet because of a lifelong fear of "bothering" anybody.

Thinking to find this idea, or similar ideas, more fully fleshed out, I'd recently read Susan Sontag's *Illness as Metaphor*. Sontag, however—with all due respect and compassion (she eventually died of breast cancer herself)—turned out to be a big, humorless crab who considered the notion of a spiritual dimension to anything to be intellectual hogwash, and had written a whole book taking the culture to task for making the entirely reasonable connection between cancer and possible death.

I didn't think cancer was a metaphor. A malignant tumor wasn't like something else; a tumor was all too grotesquely itself, which was

precisely why the knowledge that you were harboring one was so terrifying—and it must be said, so strangely compelling. Moreover, to
pinpoint the TB bacillus does not necessarily mean that the cause of
TB is "merely" physical. "Things can't go on this way," Kafka had said,
and I thought of the fear that had trapped me in drinking, in indiscriminate sex, in thinking there wouldn't be enough to go around if I
had a child.

Was it possible to have so much self-centered fear that your very
cells began to mutate? "My sickness . . . is not a real sickness," Kafka
went on to say, "but certainly cannot be called health. It belongs to
that class of illnesses which do not originate in the place where they
seem to lodge and which the doctors are even more helpless than usual
in dealing with. Of course it is the lungs, but then again it is not the
lungs."[50]

The other fascinating thing about Kafka was his sense that writing
simultaneously served to keep him alive and kill him, was both illness
(another kind of illness) and cure. He often compared writing to crucifixion—"nails pressing into the flesh,"[51] the way, beneath the desk,
"you inescapably feel the spikes in your knees,"[52]—and surely the Harrow, with its message slowly, agonizingly, inscribing itself on the body,
could also be a metaphor for the self-annihilating focus and nervous
tension required to get even a single sentence right; the way that, to
the writer, every word seems written in his or her own blood.

"God doesn't want me to write, but I—I must . . . and there's more
anguish in it than you can imagine,"[53] he remarked to one friend; and
to another, "After being lashed through periods of insanity, I began to
write, and this writing is the most important thing in the world to
me (in a way that is horrible to everyone around me, so unspeakably
horrible that I don't want to talk about it)—the way his delusion is
important to the madman (should he lose it, he would become 'mad')
or the way her pregnancy is important to a woman."[54] That Kafka had

connected writing with pregnancy was of particular interest, and again I wondered if some of us women are capable of either the vocation of motherhood or writing, but not both.

The real paradox was that by making it impossible to perform his day job as a workers' compensation lawyer (which he loathed), Kafka's TB also provided the precise conditions that fostered his work: "And so with trembling fear I protect the writing from every disturbance, and not the writing alone, but the solitude that is part of it"[55]; "Writing sustains me, but is it not more accurate to say that it sustains this [illness-dominated] way of life?"[56]

Another author whose work I admired, and who had reflected deeply upon his illness, was the late British television writer Dennis Potter. Potter had suffered from psoriatic arthropathy, a disfiguring and excruciatingly painful condition that—with the help of gargantuan quantities of alcohol, nicotine, caffeine, and morphine—had fueled a streak of creative genius. He had worn pajamas under his clothes to contain the clouds of flaking skin, turned in scripts splattered with blood and cortisone cream and, when his hand had become too crabbed with arthritis to hold a pen, strapped the pen on and continued writing anyway. Upon being diagnosed with inoperable cancer and told he had only three months to live, he had put his affairs in order and established a grueling, nonstop work schedule that had enabled him not only to finish the last two works he'd planned but also to go on and write more.

Like Kafka, Potter sensed that his illness was at least partly emotional—in his case, a manifestation of the sexual abuse he had experienced as a boy of ten—and that he may have subconsciously triggered the psoriasis himself in adult life as a release from pent-up feelings. (*The Singing Detective*, perhaps his most well-known screenplay, is based upon a character with a skin condition so severe as to confine him to a hospital bed). Also like Kafka, Potter seemed to have viewed his illness as inextricably linked to, even the driving force behind, his work. It was almost as if he had intuitively known that physical suffering would give him the solitude, the sense of apartness, and the isolation he needed to write.

Further examples of the connection between creativity and psycho-spiritual illness abounded. The poet Walt Whitman so tirelessly and heedlessly tended the Civil War wounded that he came down with an undiagnosed illness from which he never fully recovered. The emotionally delicate playwright and poet Antonin Artaud, on a return voyage by ship from Ireland (where he had traveled to deliver a walking stick he believed had belonged to St. Patrick, Satan, and Christ) had attacked a crew member, been put in a straitjacket, and spent most of the rest of his life in asylums. Simone Weil, the French intellectual, philosopher, and mystic who, in solidarity with the souls in hell refused to be baptized, had contracted TB while working for the Resistance, become further weakened by refusing to eat, and died of cardiac arrest, or anorexia, or self-starvation (to this day, no one is quite sure) in a sanitarium at the age of thirty-four.

I turned out the light and drank in the quiet of the desert. The air smelled of creosote, the wind soughed through the cottonwoods, and in their cells behind the chapel, the monks were observing the Great Silence, which lasted from Compline each night until after breakfast the next morning. I thought of the strange possibility that we can almost "invite" our diseases, of the bizarre way that the world is so often redeemed not through health and wholeness but through sickness and violence and insanity. I thought about the Incarnational mystery that all true passion is eventually worked out in and on the body. Who can plumb the depths of his or her own wounds? Who can parse out which part of our wound is killing us and which part of our wound is keeping us alive?

Maybe the reason so many writers got sick was that, bit by bit, they had ransomed their healthy flesh for stories and poems and songs. They had given every last neuron, bone-marrow cell, drop of blood to their work—leaving nothing for themselves but malignant tumors, collapsed lungs, and arteriosclerotic, patched-up hearts.

1 7

Forty Days and Forty Nights

Forty days and forty nights
You were fasting in the wild;
Forty days and forty nights
Tempted, and yet undefiled.
—George Hunt Smyttan, 1856, from a Lenten hymn

By the time I returned from St. Andrew's, I was ready to take off my bandage. The waterproof tape was starting to itch, and psychologically, I'd passed the threshold from dread to curiosity. I closed my eyes, made Tim remove the gauze, and peeked down through my fingers at my trusty breast. The flesh was bruised purple, an angry red line ran around the nipple, and though difficult to discern because of the swelling, the shape seemed ever-so-slightly off.

"At least it doesn't look like a pie with one piece gone," Tim said helpfully.

"No. More like a pillow with a little of the stuffing taken out."

My follow-up appointment with Staggers was the next day. *This is it. This is when I'm going to find out everything they know about my cancer,* I thought, gazing out the window of the ninth-story examining room wearing one of the johnnys I was starting to feel were my normal attire.

Staggers came in, with his suave manners and white lab coat, examined my incisions, said they looked good. Then, as my heart hammered in my chest, he sat down and opened my file.

"You're estrogen and progesterone positive," he began. "This is what you want, since hormone-positive tumors grow slightly more slowly than hormone-negative tumors, and they're also responsive to tamoxifen.

"The higher the reading for HER2/neu, a growth factor receptor, the more aggressive the tumor: yours is 1 on a scale of 3.

"Cancer staging is based on the size of the tumor, status of the lymph nodes, and whether or not it's metastasized. Because the lymph nodes weren't involved and the tumor was under 2 centimeters, you're a Stage 1. Cancer is also assigned a grade, based on the aggressiveness of the tumor. The lowest possible grade is 1A; yours is 1B."

This was so much news—and so much that was better than I'd dared hope—that I had trouble fully attending. Staggers, too, seemed to lack focus; in the course of delivering this pivotal (to me, anyway) information, he left the room to deal with other business not once, not twice, but three times.

"As you probably know," he continued when he returned, "one of the main characteristics of breast cancer is its unpredictability. After your treatment is finished, you might never be bothered by it again." (My heart soared.) "On the other hand, I've had patients with cases similar to yours die within six months." (I almost threw up).

He went on to say he'd met with a breast cancer "team" that morning to discuss my treatment plan. Half the folks (in the excitement of the moment, I stupidly neglected to ask how many had composed the team) had recommended radiation, four months of Adriamycin and Cytoxan (two basic types of chemo were administered to breast cancer patients: a "low-test" called CMF, and a "high-test"; this was the

high-test), and a five-year course of tamoxifen. The other half had recommended radiation and tamoxifen only.

The doctor had a good face, the face of a family man. "What would
you tell me if I were your daughter?" I asked.

"Hmm, that's a hard one," he replied. "My sister was diagnosed with
breast cancer not long ago, and she had a terrible time with chemo.
Your prognosis looks pretty good, so I might say forget the chemo; just
go with the radiation and tamoxifen."

Probably every woman asked the same question, but he'd still made
me feel, however briefly, like a person instead of a file number. When
he stood up to leave, I grasped his hand with genuine warmth.

Dealing with the fact that I could die was hard enough. But as I began
puzzling out how to think about and treat my cancer, I really did not
want to look fatally out of step. I really did not want to set myself even
further apart from the world than I already felt myself to be. I really
did not want to be thought of as crazy.

Lent, the seven-week liturgical season that starts with Ash Wednesday and culminates in Easter, had arrived. Mirroring the forty days in
the desert during which Christ was tempted by the devil, Lent was
an opportunity to get down to the bare bones and look inward. Lent
was the time to acknowledge how very much one wanted to be, for
example, famous; to look at what lay beneath one's craving for, say,
gossip and sugar; to consider that the hours frittered away playing the
fiendishly difficult computer card game Brain Jam perhaps really could
be better spent. The solutions to such temptations that rose naturally
to mind were never fasting, prayer, and giving alms. But this year the
temptation in the desert had acquired a new meaning for me. This year

the opportunity to look even more deeply inward couldn't have arrived at a more opportune time.

Ash Wednesday dawned cold and rainy. I'd decided to fast from coffee for Lent, a martyr-like sacrifice for a caffeine addict such as myself, and after six-thirty morning Mass, I decided to devote the rest of the day to meditation and prayer. Unfortunately, around eleven o'clock I also decided, for no good reason, that Tim (who had the day off) was driving me out of my mind, at which point I stormed out, took a walk in the rain, and returned only to find myself obsessed with food.

Ash Wednesday and Good Friday are days of fasting, which, according to the church's guidelines, means one full meatless meal and two smaller meals that together do not add up to one regular meal, but I had worked up such an appetite during my walk that I made a giant pan of sautéed eggplant and noodles and shortly after noon shoveled down what was supposed to be my one full meatless meal of the day and would have been an appropriate meal for a longshoreman who had not eaten in about a week.

After that I was so stuffed I had to lie down on the couch, where I stayed for most of the afternoon reading Evelyn Underhill's *Mysticism*, feeling very put upon and sorry for myself and not seeing how I could possibly go seven more weeks without coffee.

Luckily, the good Father Terry had taken it upon himself to host a series of weekly Lenten reflections, as he did every year, the first of which was to take place that very night. So after dinner I drove to the nearby offices of the L.A. Archdiocese and found my way to a bland, blue-carpeted, beige-walled room so typical of "church" the world over. Getting together with people is never my favorite activity, but these were all addicts of one kind or another—people who'd hit a hideous bottom and experienced the precarious, unlikely "resurrection" of having the obsession to drink, or go to the bathhouses, or spend or hoard money, removed. And that meant, if nothing else, that there were bound to be some laughs.

Many of the eight or ten folks in attendance I already knew: Leo, a retired Rikers Island guard; Anita, who ran a vintage clothing store; Glenn, a gay convert who was working toward a degree in marriage and family counseling. George, an artist who made sculptures from household sponges, strolled in, surveyed the company, and drawled, "So has everybody sinned today?"

There were some unfamiliar faces, too. Conny made her entrance in a silver bob, orange lipstick, and gravelly Brooklyn accent: "I don't know why he asked me to come," she kept saying, "I'm Jewish!" In fact, only a handful of us were Catholic. But to be an addict, to have been in the deadly grip of booze or anonymous sex or gambling and by some mysterious grace to have lived to tell the tale renders a person, no matter how glaring his or her continuing defects, the bearer of a strange and special light.

For my own part, to have been compelled to drink, and no longer to drink, was to have glimpsed a world way beyond this one. To be the ongoing recipient of such obviously unmerited mercy suffused every waking and sleeping moment of my better self with gratitude. That the solution to a compulsion that had very nearly killed me had turned out to be communing with a bunch of other ex-addicts and drunks—examining our blackened consciences, trying to make things right with the people we'd hurt, cracking jokes—had led me first to God and then to Christ.

Father Terry showed up carrying a gallon of cranapple juice and a stack of paperback missals. We sang (badly) a hymn, "Forty Days and Forty Nights." He talked a bit, as he often did, about his deeply alcoholic, Irish Catholic family: Uncle Matt, who used to crawl in loaded and bunk down with the kids; the father who had died at forty-two while detoxing; the sainted mother, left with five kids to raise alone, who'd been a natural theologian.

From there he segued into some remarks on fasting. The purpose of fasting, he explained, was not to punish yourself but to reveal how out of balance you tended to be. "You know you're out of balance, for example," he said, "when you go into Starbucks and you're craving that one certain muffin you like with the chocolate chips and the macadamia nuts, and the guy tells you they're out and suddenly you realize you're standing there with your voice raised an octave saying, 'But you had them yesterday!'"

His grandmother Nellie Brennan, mother of ten, Terry reported, had been generous and fun loving and had observed fasting, especially Lenten fasting, down to the letter, scrupulously measuring out her food and refusing to eat more even when she was pregnant, which may have contributed to the fact that she was the only one of Terry's four grandparents to have died before she was eighty (heeding her own mother's plea to "take the pledge," she had succumbed at the age of seventy-eight to cirrhosis of the liver, having never, in spite of the alcoholism that ran rampant through the family, taken a single drink herself).

"The danger is being neurotically obedient—obedient because you want to get spiritual good marks—but Nellie Brennan was obedient out of love," Terry said. "When obedience comes from a deep, deep faith and you're practicing it because you want to be in solidarity with Christ, man, it works. And if it hurts real bad, well then it hurts real bad, but there is a kind of joy in it."

We talked for a while about our own ideas of fasting: that you could fast not just from food but from harsh thoughts or always having to be right. We spoke of our fears: the kid in jail—again; the mother with Alzheimer's who was holding out against assisted living; the anorexic friend who was drinking nonfat salad dressing straight from the bottle. We spoke of our resentments and our desire to do a little bit better.

I could never be quite sure what, if anything, happened at these odd little gatherings: Honesty? Vulnerability? I just knew that something, imperceptibly, moved.

We sang, again very badly, a closing hymn, "The God of Love My Shepherd Is."

And in bed that night I lay awake for a long time thinking of Nellie Brennan with her ten children, fasting, and me lying on the couch all afternoon feeling sorry for myself—because I "couldn't" have a cup of coffee.

18

The Temptation to Be Relevant

Judas is neither a master of evil nor the figure of a demoniacal power of darkness but rather a sycophant who bows down before the anonymous power of changing moods and current fashion. But it is precisely this anonymous power that crucified Jesus, for it was anonymous voices that cried, "Away with him! Crucify him!" [57]

—Joseph Cardinal Ratzinger

Phase One of the cancer nightmare—the biopsy, the shock of diagnosis, surgery—was over. Phase Two, however—making a treatment decision—promised to be another major undertaking.

"You'll want to put in for an oncology consult next," had been Staggers' parting words, and they'd led to yet another unfortunate contact with the medical profession. I'd immediately schlepped down to Ricketts' office to ask in person that the request be put in as soon as possible. Dolores, apparent IQ of forty and "I care" quotient of zero, protested in her whiny nasal voice, "But we can't do anything without a note from Dr. Staggers. Dr. Staggers has to give us a note first. Dr. Ricketts can't just put in for that himself. Dr. Staggers has to fax us a note."

Two months after I'd been diagnosed with invasive breast cancer, and I was still waiting for a note to verify that I needed to see an oncologist?

Out of fear and frustration, I finally lost it. "I am so SICK of this!" I screamed at Dolores. "Why does everything have to take so insanely frickin' LONG?"

Typically, right away I felt terribly guilty and remorseful and had to call a friend or two to talk it out. I tended to keep everything bottled up and then explode, and I was also almost comically triggered by people in charge who were not (in my view) doing their job—not taking care of me. Because I so seldom asked for help, I felt that when I did ask for help, people should for God's sake help me.

I realized that people could not be expected to know my personal emotional baggage and history, and I had certainly made inroads over the years. But lack of courtesy or conscientiousness on the part of The Other made everything in me short-circuit, and after all, cancer was uncharted territory.

Later that afternoon, Ricketts himself called—for the first time since the diagnosis. "Okay," he said soothingly, "I've put an 'Urgent' on the authorization request, and meanwhile the breast cancer team has recommended—let's see . . . four months of Adriamycin and Cytoxan, six weeks of radiation, and five years of tamoxifen, to guarantee that the cancer never comes back."

Even in my untutored state I knew the word *guarantee* to be a blatant lie. And Staggers had reported that the team had in fact been split—that a full half had not recommended Adriamycin and Cytoxan at all.

As I hung up, I saw that the verdict was official: the medical profession ran exactly the same way the legal profession did: on fear, greed, apathy, and a deep desire to have as little personal interaction as possible. Parroting from my record was all Ricketts could do: as my "personal care" (a misnomer if ever there was one) physician, his entire role in the HMO scheme was to hand me off to other, equally overworked doctors. I realized that he and his staff no doubt found the system just as dehumanizing as I did, but I was starting to wonder: *Were these the folks I wanted to accompany me on one of the most emotionally fraught ordeals of my life? Were these the people to whom I wanted to entrust my body?*

I couldn't put the task off any longer: I needed to start seriously researching my treatment options. Since chemo was by far the most severe and invasive of the recommended treatments, I figured I'd start with that. *Chemo*: this was a word I had never planned on being remotely part of my life. Chemo was horrible, but chemo made you better—didn't it? Chemo was the worst, but you did chemo so you'd live—right?

I'd already found what desultory online research I'd conducted to be an exercise in frustration, and when I began looking in earnest for information on chemotherapy, I became more frustrated still. Simply plowing through the seemingly trillions of breast-cancer sites to find a piece of applicable information (with dial-up, no less—this was 2000, remember?) was a feat in itself. Then, once I did manage to find a promising page or two, trying to weasel any meaning out of the inevitable multiple sets of cross-referencing statistics would set my head spinning.

I'd come across something like, "Combined with radiation, for Stage 2, node-positive, postmenopausal women with tumors over 2 cm, one 1988 study showed that chemotherapy reduces the risk of recurrence by 28.5%." That was fine, but what if you were Stage 1, node-negative, premenopausal and with a tumor under 1 cm? What had post-1988 research shown? What were the survival rates, as opposed to the recurrence rates? Also, though I originally naively assumed that people were providing this information out of the kindness of their hearts, I eventually figured out from the fact that certain sites relentlessly pushed certain drugs that some of them perhaps had a small agenda.

Still, I didn't need to be a research expert to figure out that chemo was one gnarly treatment. I had always pictured a kind of gas chamber impregnated with toxic chemicals that got in your lungs and over your skin, but chemo was instead administered intravenously, bringing to mind lethal injections and therefore making the prospect seem somehow even creepier.

As opposed to radiation—a local treatment that killed cancer cells only in the breast—chemo was a systemic therapy which treated the whole body by interfering with the process of cell division. Because the chemicals worked on all rapidly dividing cells, they unfortunately killed not only cancer cells but also hair cells, intestinal-wall cells, and bone marrow cells as well. Consequently, head hair fell out; eyebrows, eyelashes, pubic hair, leg and arm hair fell out; and in many cases, fingernails and toenails fell off. Adriamycin, which Staggers had recommended for me, could "leak out of the vein and cause a very severe burn that could require skin grafting," according to Dr. Love.[58] Nausea and vomiting for up to two days after the treatment were common. Chemo caused hot flashes and regularly induced menopause in premenopausal women.

You could die from chemo. In *The Cancer Industry*, Dr. Ralph W. Moss had written:

> The bone marrow is the foundation of the immune system, which seems to serve the dual function of preventing infections and combating the spread of cancer. The use of chemotherapy is often accompanied by destruction of this immune system. Chemotherapy often brings in its train a host of blood-deficiency diseases. . . . These, in turn, can give rise to massive, uncontrollable infections. Cancer patients on chemotherapy have been known to die of something as innocuous as the common cold.[59]

But what really floored me was that chemo didn't even do that much good, especially—though the medical profession relentlessly pushed it anyway—for early Stage 1 patients like me. "Chemotherapy reduces the risk of recurrence by about a third. That means the higher the chance of recurrence the larger the difference that chemotherapy will make for you. . . . [I]f your chance of recurrence is 9 percent, like the average node-negative woman with a tumor less than two centimeters, [chemo] will improve it by 3 percent," Dr. Love observed.[60]

Buried in the statistics was one more shocking fact: contrary to what I'd always believed, even when chemo "worked," that usually meant two or three extra years, not the rest of your "natural" life.[61] The possibility of dying versus a reduction in the chance of recurrence from 9% to 6%—or, since my tumor was smaller than one centimeter, an even more negligible reduction? Two or three extra years, and for at least one of them I'd be sick as a dog?

I couldn't believe that a mere few weeks ago I'd been saying that I wanted them to throw every treatment in the book at me, that I was going to demand chemo. I wasn't saying at this stage of the game I'd refuse chemo, but I was certainly going to give some very serious consideration to the pros and cons.

I called a breast-cancer advocacy center in Berkeley and spoke to a woman who told me that I should take as long as I needed, that to feel comfortable with my decision was of paramount importance, and that a month or two wasn't going to make much difference. She also said that statistics had their place but that they really couldn't tell you much, if anything, about your particular disease. Breast cancer was a very complex illness with innumerable factors, some of which weren't even known, she said, and therefore everyone's case was completely different.

If everyone was completely different, I wondered as I hung up, why did they push everyone to have almost the exact same treatment?

I was starting to realize that more than cancer was at stake: I was facing huge questions about how I wanted to live from now on and, possibly, how to die. As if on cue, suddenly I was bombarded with information about the less-than-morally-pristine universe of health care. I read in the newspaper that the prestigious *New England Journal of Medicine* had been exposed in several blatant conflict-of-interest situations with pharmaceutical companies. I heard on a public radio slot that contrary to the study results—many, if not all, of which turned out to have been falsified—the painful, expensive bone-marrow transplants doctors had been performing on metastatic breast-cancer patients did not improve survival rates at all.

And on a more immediate front, every morning I sat across the table from Tim and listened to tales of his harrowing night at work at a sprawling teaching hospital that was a major dumping ground for L.A.'s uninsured: the homeless, the mentally ill, the illegal immigrants. Up until now his stories—the terminal AIDS patients having their thousandth sample of blood drawn; the people with clearly fatal brain tumors on whom the doctors were still performing useless surgeries—had seemed depressing but abstract. Now such practices were revealed in their true light as horrifying. "Why can't the poor patients be left alone?" I asked him. "Why can't they be placed in hospice and die in peace?"

"They give the doctors a chance to practice," he said, averting his eyes, "plus the hospital's afraid of getting sued for failing to take every possible measure." I thought of the people who self-righteously blathered about leaving a "small carbon footprint" but thought nothing of taking torturous, life-prolonging measures that cost the health-care system, insurance companies (not that I cared about them), taxpayers, and in the end all of us millions upon millions of dollars. I thought of my father's death the summer before: the way the doctors had pumped antibiotics into him way past the point when everyone knew they couldn't do any good; our own reluctance to take him off the dialysis that was technically keeping him alive.

Modern medicine had created a set of impossible questions, and I wondered, as I would many times in the coming months, which was worse: to die sooner rather than later, as people had in the "old days," or to be shored up over and over again, only to suffer incremental but ever-increasing losses—to linger indefinitely, on an alien hospital bed, in loneliness and pain.

19

The Thin Line between Passion and Pathology

Strive always to prefer, not that which is easiest, but that which is most difficult;
Not that which is most delectable, but that which is most unpleasing;
Not that which gives most pleasure, but rather that which gives least;
Not that which is restful, but that which is wearisome;
Not that which is consolation, but rather that which is disconsolateness;
Not that which is greatest, but that which is least;
Not that which is loftiest and most precious, but that which is lowest and most despised;
Not that which is a desire for anything, but that which is a desire for nothing;
Strive to go about seeking not the best of temporal things, but the worst.
Strive thus to desire to enter into complete detachment and emptiness and poverty,
with respect to everything that is in the world, for Christ's sake.[62]

—St. John of the Cross, *Ascent of Mount Carmel*

A couple of years earlier, I'd started seeing a pixie-ish woman with a head of short, graying curls and turned-out feet in church around the 'hood and at Mass at St. Basil's. She wore vaguely bohemian clothes—berets, embroidered peasant blouses—and her smile was so brilliant that I hardly noticed the one tooth missing in her left lower jaw and the line of brown that ran along the tops of the rest. One morning after Mass she tapped me on the shoulder and said, "You wouldn't want a little black puppy, would you?"

Her name, it turned out, was Barbara, and when she invited me over to the run-down house she rented in the Hispanic ghetto of Pico-Union a week or so later, I learned that she was a sort of ambassadress to the halt and lame of the animal kingdom. From a yard of packed dirt, a ragtag menagerie of cats and dogs bayed and meowed and hurled themselves against Barbara's legs. A leprous collie sported a sweater fashioned from the lining of a Burberry raincoat; a litter of mangy kittens lounged on a scrap of claw-ripped Astroturf; and a one-eyed German shepherd, front legs tucked into the sleeves of a quilted blue parka, frolicked with a tailless tabby.

"How many animals do you have?" I asked, trying to bat away the snout of a Dalmatian with a cast on his leg who was trying to mount me.

"Nine dogs and fifteen cats—Cut that out, Minnie!—but that's not counting the strays."

Pets were one ministry, but Barbara's true calling was dance. Six days a week, she rose at 4:00 a.m. to take care of the animals, schlepped on foot the mile to St. Basil's for 6:25 Mass, and took an hour-and-a-half-one-way bus ride to Studio City in the San Fernando Valley for ballet lessons. Barbara didn't dance for money or recognition or success but as a form of prayer: "I offer my body—my pain and sweat—to someone who needs it more than me," she matter-of-factly reported. She'd had the same teacher for thirty years.

"Thirty years!" I said. "The two of you must be joined at the hip by now!"

"Just the opposite," she laughed. "Technical proficiency is important, of course, but more important to me is the willingness to grow organically as a dancer, the inner knowledge that takes a lifetime to cultivate. Because I allow myself to look awkward in order to, for example, really feel how my shoulders are connected to my back, I'm ostracized by the other students and mercilessly ridiculed by my teacher."

Barbara was entirely unconcerned with adequate sleep, decent food, or, beyond *Prairie Home Companion* on Saturday nights and an occasional episode of *Frasier* (she liked the dog), leisure. In her free time she practiced at the makeshift barre in her apartment—one Hail Mary for every plié—ran errands for her senile Russian landlady Henrietta, did laundry, hauled home sacks of kitty litter from Smart & Final, trekked around picking up more strays, and made endless trips to the vet, all by foot or bus. Her joints had begun to tighten up—she'd just turned fifty—which meant a half-hour of exercises when she got out of bed each morning simply to be able to walk.

To me, her existence seemed like one long punishment; to her, it was evidently heaven. "I feel like I'm running a marathon," she said, her eyes lighting up. "Every day a new challenge."

"Aren't you tired all the time?" I asked her. "Don't you ever want a break?"

"I didn't start out like this," she replied. "My way of being evolved over time. When you're on a spiritual path, you have to make sacrifices. You have to get smaller so God can get bigger. You have to more or less offer up . . ."

"Your whole life?" I asked hesitantly.

"Yeah," she replied.

Barbara was an affront to every civilized notion of success, health, security, and mainstream religious belief, and the more I saw of her, the more I decided she was possibly more like Christ, or at least John the Baptist, than anyone I had ever met. *Is she crazy?* I kept wondering, but truly crazy people don't know they're crazy. Barbara knew she was weird.

"Some people would call me masochistic for sticking with my teacher," she'd say, "but to me, the fact that he's difficult is an opportunity to grow." Or "People ask, 'Why do you spend so much money on animals? You should be helping humans.' But one doesn't have to be at the expense of the other. You can't believe the things I learn about people, for example, by living with animals: one needs to be on a leash; another can't get along with his neighbors; a third is sick and needs lots of love. And because I allow myself to be interrupted at all hours to nurse and walk and rescue them, I'm forced to be faithful in a way that, left to my own devices, I never would have been."

Maybe, I thought, *and maybe you're also a pathological animal hoarder* (a bit of a hoarder myself—food, money—I'd researched this scary condition and found the symptoms fit Barbara almost to a T). Still, her way of life fascinated me, and whenever we got together for coffee at the local Mexican bakery, I plied her with questions.

All institutions and organizations filled Barbara with scorn. She rejected social workers as paid professionals, was virulently antigovernment (when I once asked whether she collected welfare, she replied, aghast, "Oh God, no. I wouldn't have anything to do with the state"), and disdained charities. "They have their hand out for AIDS research, but do you think those people would help *you* if you were poor?" she railed. "No, it's 'Give us a hundred dollars for a shot; give us a thousand dollars for a month's worth of pills, and we'll help you!' Otherwise, you could die in the street for all they care."

I suppose I shouldn't have been surprised when Barbara also expressed less than unalloyed regard for modern medicine. "Every time you have a little pain, take an aspirin, they tell you! But you never grow that way, you never learn anything! That's why I don't trust doctors. Their only goal is to avoid pain! Their biggest fear is death!"

"Well, shouldn't it be?" I asked warily.

"No!" she replied. "As money is to the material world, suffering is to the spiritual world. We have no idea of the value of suffering."

Barbara, it turned out, had a very highly developed notion of suffering. She believed that the suffering of animals somehow relieved ours. She believed we could and should take the burden upon ourselves to suffer for others. "You know that passage in the Gospel where the woman who's been hemorrhaging for twelve years touches the hem of Christ's garment and is healed?" she asked (Luke 8:40–56). "Have you ever noticed which story immediately follows? It's the story of the little girl who dies and is brought back to life by Christ. And how old is the child? Twelve! Do you see? It's almost as if the woman had been keeping the child alive with her suffering."

Barbara was so hard-core, in fact, that she didn't even believe in dentists—which explained that missing tooth.

"Same as doctors," she said. "They're all about avoiding pain and making everybody pretty. Everybody's so afraid not to look pretty!"

Oddly enough, Barbara was extremely pretty herself, but I had to admire her consistency. Other people were sympathetic, embarrassed, and appalled when I broke the news that I had cancer. Barbara, I swear, was jealous.

"Look at St. Thérèse of Lisieux! She was thrilled when she started coughing up blood! Look at St. Bernadette, who had a giant tumor on her leg and never told a soul. Other people would have moped around feeling sorry for themselves, but sickness filled them with joy!"

"You mean if you knew you had cancer, you wouldn't even see a doctor?" I asked.

"No, no, no, I wouldn't let a doctor touch me. Do what's right for you; go the normal route if you have to; but do whatever you decide to do with joy. People are going to be watching, and you can be an example; you can help them not be quite so afraid if they get sick. Show them something new; teach them something. Be creative even in death. Make illness an opportunity to demonstrate God's love. Turn your suffering around. Use the very weapon that's being used against you to create. Use the anxiety you're feeling to stay up all night writing. Look at what all those composers and poets and saints who died young accomplished in a very short period of time."

As usual, rejection slips were pouring over the transom, and what with the pitiful tragedy that had befallen me, I was starting to feel that the time had come for a well-deserved break. But talking to Barbara, I was reminded of how, in the essay collection *Mystery and Manners*, Flannery O'Connor had observed that most people are not interested in writing but in being a "writer" and making money; that nobody has any business writing unless he or she has the gift of a calling; that a gift is a considerable responsibility requiring sacrifice, discipline, and asceticism.

I remembered that, swollen with cortisone, her joints crippled with lupus, she had hidden stories under the pillow of her hospital bed to revise when the nurses weren't looking. I remembered that when her mother urged her to go to Lourdes and pray for a cure, she had gone only reluctantly, saying that she would rather be able to write than walk. I remembered Hulga from "Good Country People" and the Misfit from "A Good Man Is Hard to Find" and Mrs. Turpin from "Revelation"—characters whose stories I had read so many times that they were more real to me than many people I actually knew—and I thought with a stab of gratitude what it had cost her to get the stories right.

And then I slunk to my desk, turned on the computer, and got down to work.

20

The Seed Is in Darkness

We are the soil of the divine seed; there is no other. The flowering of Christ in us does not depend upon pious exercises, on good works outside our daily life, on an amateur practice of religion in our leisure time. It is in the marrow of our bones, in the experience of our daily life.
The seed is in darkness: the darkness of sorrow, the darkness of faith.[63]

—Caryll Houselander

Staggers had recommended that I take tamoxifen for the next five years, so I figured I'd research that next. Recently hailed as a kind of hormonal therapy wonder drug, the nutshell description was that too much estrogen contributed to breast cancer; tamoxifen blocked estrogen and thereby supposedly prevented the growth of new tumors.

The whole area of estrogen vis-à-vis breast cancer, however, was very confusing. If estrogen was harmful, didn't reason dictate that estrogen-positive tumors would be more dangerous than those that were estrogen-negative? But no: "In general, tumors that are sensitive to hormones—that have receptors—are slightly slower growing and have a slightly better prognosis than tumors that aren't," Dr. Love said.[64] And while I would have guessed that an estrogen blocker would be even more effective on estrogen-negative tumors that didn't attract much estrogen in the first place, in fact, tamoxifen worked only on women whose tumors were estrogen-positive, as mine was.

The confusion was reflected, among other places, in the controversy that swirled around estrogen replacement therapy. "It used to be felt that women with breast cancer could never take hormones because it would be 'like pouring gasoline on a fire' and would immediately cause the cancer to flare up," Dr. Love wrote. "Recently the trend of putting all women on postmenopausal hormones has led us to reevaluate this premise. Physicians are noting that there are no data and have done a 180-degree switch. We used to say, 'No data so don't take it.' Now we are saying, 'No data so it's okay.'"[65]

This casual reversal of stance struck me as especially alarming in light of Dr. Love's admission that "tamoxifen is a very peculiar drug. In some ways it blocks estrogen, as it does in the breast, but in other organs like the liver, bones, and uterus, it acts like estrogen."[66] In other words, while decreasing the rate of recurrence for breast cancer, tamoxifen promoted cancer of the liver and uterus. No big deal, most doctors said to the upsurge in uterine cancer; just have a hysterectomy.

Others weren't so sanguine. In the opinion of researcher, author, and cancer expert/establishment gadfly Samuel Epstein, for example, tamoxifen was "an extremely dangerous drug," the side effects of which included blood clots, depression, and weight gain. It tripled the risk of uterine cancer, and it was "one of the most potent known liver carcinogens, making it likely that a significant number of healthy women receiving Tamoxifen will die from liver cancer within a decade or so, without any warning of this very grave risk."[67]

As to effectiveness, according to Epstein, there was no hard evidence that tamoxifen reduced the rates of breast cancer at all,[68] and even the conservative Dr. Love admitted, "At this point it is still not clear that, in premenopausal women [tamoxifen] adds anything to chemotherapy or works as well as an adjuvant treatment."[69]

On the contrary, manipulating a system so complex that nobody really knew how it worked could apparently have some unintended, and alarming, consequences. The authors of *Tamoxifen and Breast Cancer*, for example, described research showing that though tamoxifen initially blocks estrogen in the body, thereby causing breast cancer tumors to shrink, whatever cancer cells remained eventually learn to *thrive* on the drug.[70]

Martin Tenniswood, Notre Dame's Coleman Professor of Biology, had come to a similar conclusion. An article in *Notre Dame Magazine* reported: "Tamoxifen kills most but not all the tumor cells. . . . In those cells that don't die, it appears the drug backfires causing them to produce substances that induce cell survival and also an enzyme that 'chews up' material around the cell. Normally dying cells produce the enzyme causing the tumor to shrink. When surviving cells produce it, trouble results. Metastatic cancer cells, the most dangerous form which spread throughout the body, produce high levels of this enzyme. . . . It allows them to invade other tissue. 'The drug may not be as good a preventative as we thought,' Tenniswood concluded. 'It may result in the woman developing a more aggressive form of breast cancer later on.'"[71]

None of this exactly made me want to jump in the tamoxifen sign-up line. The prospect of contracting a kind of revenge-bent killer strain of breast cancer sometime in the future gave me real pause, as did the fact that I found tamoxifen, and the way it was marketed and promoted, uncomfortably reminiscent of the Pill.

To wit, in the sixties, the medical gods had been only too glad to announce, Oh look, here's something to make life easier, a handy little birth-control tablet! Only thirty years later were they were discovering that the higher the number of periods a woman has throughout her lifetime, the higher the estrogen level and the higher the corresponding risk of breast cancer. Only thirty years later were they discovering, in other words, that the Pill had side effects that hadn't been initially foreseen. Everyone assumed unlimited choice was a good thing, but to me this was only one of the many ways in which the unlimited "choices" of modern life were actually killing us.

Then I happened upon a piece in *The New Yorker* by the writer Malcolm Gladwell (before he became a household name) entitled "John Rock's Error: What the Co-inventor of the Pill Didn't Know: Menstruation Can Endanger Women's Health."[72]

According to Gladwell, the Pill had been developed by a supposedly staunch Catholic who, to appease the Catholic hierarchy and cater to what he perceived to be women's desires, had touted the Pill as "natural" and had unnecessarily "built in" menstrual periods to its cycle.

The Church had seen through the ruse and refused to condone the Pill; Rock had died in obscurity, bitterly lapsed. What got me was that Gladwell made this out—the fact that Rock had "allowed" women to still have periods—to be his fatal error. Gladwell's idea was that if only women had taken the Pill and also had their periods artificially shut down, everything would have been great: they would have been free from the pesky risk of unwanted pregnancy, and because their estrogen levels would have been kept low, they wouldn't have been getting breast cancer either. His solution for us women now, accordingly, was to develop another, stronger pill that would manipulate our hormonal systems to the point that we would stop menstruating altogether.

I could hardly believe there had not been a nationwide uprising against such a corrupt, hateful, and antihuman idea. This is where our so-called revolutionary women's movement had brought us; this was what passed in contemporary culture for enlightened progress. We were getting breast cancer from the pill they told us was going to set us free, and to set us free from the fear of breast cancer, we were going to take another pill. We were poised to blindly welcome yet another anonymous technological/pharmaceutical invasion—proposed by a man, of course—into the most sacred, private part of our lives.

Sometimes I felt as if I were trying to do the impossible, which was to live "apart" from the world, as every writer must in one way or another, but with no real spiritual or emotional intimate. I wondered whether I was truly willing to make whatever sacrifices I was being called to, or whether I was just an ingrate malcontent trying to give my actions some other, more rarefied label.

But I sometimes thought, *What if Jesus came along right now? Would I recognize him? Would I have time for him?* And in a weird way, I thought I probably would. In a way, I was always on the lookout for him. I seemed to have nothing "better to do" than wait for him. Enough money came in to live on, like the miracle of the loaves and fishes (not that I didn't work my tail off for it). I was busy but not overcrowded. I was occupied but waiting, and I was waiting, but I was also ready. Like one of the wise virgins in the parable of the wise and foolish virgins (Matthew 25:1–13), my lamp was more or less in oil.

Consequently, I "saw" Christ all the time: in myself, in the poor and the rich, in my friends. All day long my phone rang, with people saying in so many words, How can I take the beam out of my eye before taking the splinter out of my neighbor's eye? Or, Check it out; I actually managed for once to refrain from throwing the first stone! Or, I so want to get off my mat and walk, but I can't! Those friends kept me alive. They were all I had. They were why I wrote, why I lived. Religion for me wasn't a possession I appropriated to my own ends. It was the fabric of my life, my very flesh and lifeblood, the quenching of my ravening hunger and slavering thirst.

One day around this time, my friend Ron—a film buff, journalist, and musicologist who drove an incredibly dented Civic—made a brilliant observation. He said that when he got clean and discovered he had hepatitis C from shooting drugs, he was glad, glad for all of it.

Getting clean and getting hep C both showed that actions have consequences, that what we do matters.

For some reason, this simple thought struck me as revelatory; I mulled it over for days. Believing in a world free from consequences was the biggest temptation of all. Do this and you won't feel guilty. Do that and no one will know. Quell those gnawing existential questions about being, doing, making, loving, with a pill, a drug, a surgical "procedure." Consume, spend, litter, genetically engineer, believe yourself to be the center of the universe, let technology rule your body, and suffer no repercussions. But all those things were impossible, and if they were possible, the world would be a place of infinitely more suffering than already existed. If actions didn't have consequences, no good, eternal-fruit consequences would follow from good actions. The world wouldn't only be fallen; the world would be irredeemable.

If my own actions had contributed to my illness—and of course I would never know—that didn't mean that breast cancer was a judgment, only that actions have consequences. Cancer aside, the evil wasn't so much that I had drank and smoked, slept around, had abortions, and used men and myself as objects. The evil was that I had settled for so long, in every area of my life, for the shortcut instead of the slower, more arduous path of changing my behavior, awakening consciousness, and growth.

I talked tamoxifen over with Tim, and the more I pondered, the less attractive five years of it seemed. Chemo seemed scarier by the moment too. I was going way out on a limb now—farther, even if only in my thoughts, than I'd ever imagined. What I was considering might be totally crazy, but around the edges of my brain I was starting to wonder: Could I possibly get by with just radiation?

21

Strong Meat

*To do all I can for others and for the good of souls, to take refuge
often in my "inner cell" to pray, to adore, and to unite myself to
the beloved Master. To make of everything—all prayer, suffering,
self-denial, and action—an interior offering for others and for
God's glory, as well as for those I love.*[73]
—Servant of God Elisabeth Leseur

With visions of Nellie Brennan floating in my mind's eye, I'd thought
a lot about fasting over the last few weeks: thought about it but, other
than giving up coffee and cutting back on sugar, not done a whole lot
about it. Pray, fast, give alms, Christ had said. He had fasted for forty
days, but even going without breakfast was a fast for me.

I have always loved food—shopping for food, reading about food,
cooking food, eating food. As a matter of fact, one of the main reasons
I had never been able to leave L.A. was that I couldn't bear to think of
giving up such a cornucopia of great, cheap food: the Monterey Park
noodle joints, the dim sum palaces, the garlic chicken at Zankou's, the
roast pork at the Cuban restaurant Versailles, the Armenian markets in
East Hollywood, Noshi Sushi. Loving food per se wasn't wrong, but
it occurred to me that there might be something wrong with making
certain kinds of it so much a part of your identity that you weren't sure
you could exist without them. To transform my approach to food, I
began to see, would be to transform everything.

One Monday morning in the parking lot of St. Basil's, I ran into Sean Dolan, a seventyish Irishman who looked like the angel in *It's a Wonderful Life*, had been sober for years, and was squiring a fellow with a ratlike face who was clearly coming off a major bender. Sean was one of these hearty cradle Catholics who is always going off to Europe to visit shrines and talking about some miracle or other. He'd once lent me a very good book called *Abandonment to Divine Providence*, by an eighteenth-century priest named Jean Pierre de Caussade. I liked Sean.

Still, when he asked about my cancer and, right there in the parking lot, grabbed my arm and said, "Come here, let's pray," I instinctively recoiled. In New England, where I come from, even your own parents don't hug you, and I had never quite grown used to the touchy-feely ways of Southern Californians. But Sean got a hold of me, and then he made the hungover guy, who reeked of booze, come over, and we all put our arms around each other, and Sean placed his free hand on the upper part of my chest and started pouring out a very heartfelt prayer. "Jesus, we ask you to help Heather," he said, with just a hint of a brogue. "You know she loves you SO MUCH, and we ask you to heal her: every tissue, every cell, every limb, every organ."

Ten years ago—okay, one year ago—I would have died of embarrassment to be standing out in public praying with a geriatric Irish Catholic and some poor mangy drunk, but the great thing about having cancer is that situations that formerly might have seemed traumatic pale in comparison. Also, you very quickly realize you can no longer afford to scoff at anybody who might even remotely have the capacity, and more to the point, willingness, to help.

After a few seconds I realized that to be embraced by these kind, well-meaning folks, who no doubt had many better things to do than take time out of their busy morning to comfort me, actually felt good. So afterward, I said, "Wow, Sean, I sure am glad we ran into each other!" and shook the rat-faced guy's hand, and we went our separate ways with smiles, waves, and on my part at least, a warm glow of gratitude.

Everything was fine until around two the next morning, when I got up to use the bathroom and thought, *That's strange, I could swear I'm feeling a little nauseous.* Within thirty minutes I was alternately retching over the toilet bowl and evacuating my bowels and did not stop for the next eighteen hours. Every twenty minutes I'd get up, crawl to the bathroom, bring up the few pitiful swallows of soda water I'd managed to down in the interim, and stagger back to the couch to lie like a whimpering animal, waiting to be overcome by the next bout. The upshot was that, through no virtue of my own but because I was too busy being deathly ill, I went an entire day without eating.

I woke the following morning feeling fit as a fiddle. Tim insisted the problem had been food poisoning, but we'd eaten the same things all day, so if that were the case, why hadn't he gotten sick too? Another, more startling, theory occurred to me. Could the fact that right after Sean performed his "laying on of hands" I'd undergone a bodily purge have been sheer coincidence? What could it mean that I had prayed for healing and immediately been struck with an illness that, for the next twenty-four hours, made eating impossible?

This was a line of reasoning I knew only Barbara could appreciate, so that night I gave her a call. Not only did she instantly see the connection, but she herself had been fasting all through Lent: every Friday and Monday she had a cup of coffee in the morning and a couple of glasses of OJ during the day and didn't eat till ten at night. "I have a book you might like," she further informed me and, after Mass the next Sunday, produced from her cat-hair-covered carpetbag a musty paperback called *The Miracle of Fasting.*

"Life-extension specialist" Paul C. Bragg, the author of this fascinating tome, had apparently enjoyed a heyday in the mid-1950s. The cover bore a photo of a Nordic-looking chap with a blinding smile, glowing skin, and a head of wavy blond hair. Inside were several more author photos: Paul against a backdrop of virile tropical plants ("Paul C. Bragg, World's Leading Healthy Lifestyle Authority")[74]; Paul in a bare-chested fighter's stance and toothy grin, sporting a pair of lederhosen ("The Bragg System of *Super Power Breathing* Built Bragg a Powerful, Healthy Body")[75]; Paul with a microscope and a pile of fruit ("Scientific Fasting Explained").[76]

Scattered throughout the book in boldface were gems of the Paul C. Bragg philosophy—"WHY NOT ENJOY LIFE TO 120?"[77]; "SICKNESS IS A CRIME—DON'T BE A CRIMINAL"[78]; "LIFE CAN BE A HAPPY AND JOYOUS ADVENTURE"[79]—and accounts of the amazing triumphs he had scored through fasting.

A typical feat was the time Paul set out to prove that contrary to popular belief, salt is not needed during extremely hot weather. He'd gone to Death Valley in the middle of July, hired ten husky young college athletes to make the trek with him, and hiked—skipped, almost—the thirty miles from Furnace Creek to Stovepipe Wells. The college boys had drunk cola and eaten ham-and-cheese sandwiches and salt tablets. Paul, of course, had fasted. By four in the afternoon, the last of the athletes had "collapsed in the hot burning sun and had to be rushed back to the ranch for medical care."[80]

Paul, on the other hand, "felt fresh as a daisy! I was not full of salt tablets and I was not full of food because I was on a complete fast. The college boys wanted cold water, but I drank only pure distilled water, not chilled. I finished the 30 mile hike in around 10 ½ hours and I had no ill effects whatsoever!"[81]

As Tim said, "Well, his name's appropriate." Still, the potential for physical, emotional, and spiritual healing through fasting suddenly electrified me. What could be more brilliant: a remedy that didn't cost anything, was at your fingertips every moment, and hurt? Not that there was any benefit to pain for its own sake, but letting part of your identity and attachments die had to hurt a little. You had to die before you could live.

The next Friday, for the first time in my life, I voluntarily had nothing to eat or drink (save a few glasses of lemon juice and water with a little maple syrup mixed in) until dinner. Going without food was hard, but around noon, when the hunger pangs had dulled to an ache, I began in a way to like the feeling of emptiness. I realized how automatically and instantly every want of mine was usually filled. I thought of how millions, possibly billions, of people were going hungry that day through no choice of their own. I came to a place of quiet and thankfulness and prayer.

The next morning I woke feeling clean, fresh, and rested. Paul C. Bragg—for perhaps slightly different reasons than mine—would have been proud.

Meanwhile, practically every article I had read on breast-cancer prevention mentioned the apparent connection between a high incidence of breast cancer and a high-fat diet. I'd been laboring under the misapprehension that my diet was relatively low-fat already, but on my next trip to the grocery store I started examining those little labels to which I'd never before paid the slightest attention, and I was staggered by what I found. I couldn't believe how much fat was in one serving of cheese—which, by the way, consisted of a mere inch cube.

Who in their right mind had ever been satisfied with only a cubic inch of cheese? Eggs, ice cream, and butter—my beloved bread without my beloved butter?—were also major offenders. Olives and nuts unfortunately were also loaded with fat. Weren't you supposed to have some fat, I started wondering. Wouldn't you die otherwise—of grief, if nothing else?

Over the course of the next couple of weeks, I read *A Cancer Battle Plan* and *The Breast Cancer Prevention Diet*. I read the "cleansing diet schedule" from a place called Health Quarters Lodge. I read about toxic diet, toxic dentistry, and toxic emotions. I read about the healing power of juice fasting, the effect of sugar intake on phagocytosis, the importance of an acid/alkaline balance. I read about macrobiotics, Laetrile, Vitamin C, and hydrogen sulfate.

After I had read enough books and talked to enough people, I became thoroughly confused. One book said to drink flax seed oil, and another said to more or less subsist on flax meal. One book said to eat nothing but brown rice and seaweed; another said to eat nothing but fruits and vegetables, and one man who had cured himself of supposedly fatal lung cancer told me that under no circumstances should you eat any fruit at all because sugar feeds cancer. Every breast-cancer diet book I read said you should practically live on soy, but after I'd been shoveling down tofu and edamame by the vatful for a few days, I spoke to a friend of a friend who said her acupuncturist had told her that soy was good for other types of cancer, but in the case of breast cancer should be avoided at all costs. One person said to buy seventy-five bucks worth of Essiac tea, which had been developed by a Canadian nurse from a formula used by the Ojibway people, and another person said Essiac tea was a big hoax and to try ginkgo.

Many of the alternative diets seemed to be based on superstition: a glass of carrot juice at ten, a dish of grated beets at eleven, any deviation from which could be fatal. That's when I decided I was not going to get too worked up about diet. Cutting down on sugar and fat and coffee and meat (and everything else that made life worth living) had to help, and I'd already decided to fast every Friday until dinner. But I knew that if I got too fanatical, every "slip" would stress me out so badly I might as well start scarfing Valrhona truffles and crème fraîche three times a day.

More to the point, I was coming to see that whether you were physically healed or not, the real point was spiritual healing—which had to be available to everybody. The answer couldn't be purchasing a black-walnut fungus that cost eighty-five dollars an ounce or flying to some Swiss clinic where you get your colon irrigated every five minutes. In fact, many of the breast-cancer diet experts had come to the conclusion that what led to a lower incidence of breast cancer wasn't so much less fat as fewer calories in general.

That insatiable consumerism could kill not only metaphorically but literally; that optimum health, personally and collectively, would be generated by eating only when and what I needed—not using food as a stab at filling the existential void with "pleasure"—only made sense. What seemed way more important than following the letter of any particular diet was learning to treat food as part of the continuum of the sacrament of life. Thus, first, last, and always, the Eucharist.

In the end, maybe the most radical change in my eating habits was this: when Tim and I sat down to dinner each night, I started saying grace.

22

Hiroshima Notes

What happened in Hiroshima twenty years ago was an absurdly horrendous massacre; but it may be the first harbinger of the world's real end, in which the human race as we know it will be succeeded by beings with blood and cells so ruined that they cannot be called human. The most terrifying monster lurking in the darkness of Hiroshima is precisely the possibility that man might become no longer human.[82]

—Kenzaburo Oe, *Hiroshima Notes*

I'd been thinking of radiation as a walk in the park compared to chemo, almost fun. But when I consulted *Dr. Susan Love's Breast Book*, the chapter began, "The idea of radiation therapy may make you nervous. After all, radiation can cause cancer, and the last thing you want is to find yourself in danger of even more cancer."[83]

Reading on, I found that, far from being a breezy little lark, radiation had side effects that included asymptomatic rib fractures; a "sunburn" effect; tiredness ("The body seems to be using all its resources to cope with the radiation, and doesn't leave much energy for anything else. . . . The fatigue may last several months after the treatment has finished, or may even begin after the course of treatment is over");[84] lung damage ("Depending on how your chest is built, a little of the radiation may get to your lung and give you a cough");[85] thickened darker-colored skin; crusty nipples [dear Lord!] that took up to six months to heal; swelling and sensitivity; depression; compounding of the scarring from surgery; increased risk of lymphedema; problems with the nerves that go from the arm to the hand, causing numbness to the fingertips [this was thankfully rare]; costochondritis, a kind of arthritis that caused inflammation of the space between the breasts where the rib and breastbone connect ("The pain can be scary—you wonder if your cancer has spread");[86] and a permanent change in the feel of the breast ("It will never feel completely normal again: you'll continue to have some sharp, shooting pains from time to time—how often varies greatly from woman to woman").[87]

Finally, Staggers had neglected to mention one major fact: because radiation above a certain dosage damaged normal tissue, a breast could tolerate only a single round; if a second lump appeared, the only option (in the eyes of the medical profession) would be a mastectomy.

Somehow radiation didn't sound quite so innocuous after that. Although it had been shown to reduce by 20 percent to 30 percent the chance of recurrence in the breast, as with chemo, if my chance was only 9 percent to begin with, was risking all those side effects worth reducing the chance to, say, 7 percent? Also, I started thinking, what about Madame Curie and all those women in the forties who had painted glow-in-the-dark radium numbers on watches, licked the tips of their paintbrushes, and started dying off like flies? What about the *MAMM* article pointing out that because radiation makes cells mutate, some doctors believed mammograms could cause, as well as detect, breast cancer? Weren't the people who invented radiation essentially the same folks who brought us Nagasaki? Did I really want to microwave my breast?

One facet of Dr. Love's chapter on radiation I found extremely odd: in spite of all the information on recurrence rates, she was silent as to what extent, if any, radiation improved one's chances of surviving. It turned out there was a very good reason for this. After hours of online research, I learned that radiation had no discernible effect on breast cancer survival rates.[88]

How could this be? If there were less chance of a second lump appearing in the breast, didn't common sense dictate that the cells from the (presumably prevented) second tumor would never have a chance to move into the lymph nodes, spread throughout the body, and metastasize, and that the survival rate would therefore rise? If you killed the cells in the breast, was the original cancer more likely to simply metastasize somewhere else? Did radiation reduce the risk of local recurrence but increase the chance, if the cancer did recur, that it would kill you? Did deaths from side effects wipe out the benefits?

Whatever the case, why run all those risks and not even improve your long-term chances? And, more to the point, why didn't the jokers tell you right up front?

I had always dismissed conspiracy theorists as airheaded nutcakes, but the more I thought about the way tumors eventually learned to thrive on tamoxifen, and the mystery of how radiation could kill cancer cells in the breast but not improve survival rates, and the way the medical profession told you next to absolutely nothing, the more I began to think that maybe conspiracy theorists didn't go far enough.

It was as if a spiritual law-of-the-universe metaphor applied to each of the proposed treatments. Chemo was like a reverse parable of the tares and the wheat (Matthew 13:24–30): instead of letting the bad grow up with the good and sorting things out later, chemo cut both the bad and the good off at the root, thereby laying devastation to the whole crop.

Radiation demonstrated the spiritual axiom that you can't turn something against others (the "others" here being the noncancerous cells of your own body) without turning it against yourself.

As for tamoxifen, the fact almost seemed to be that fighting evil with more evil—with anything less than love—only forced the evil to manifest in another form. Nothing illustrated this more clearly than our violent, hate-based culture. We kept executing criminals and manufacturing nuclear weapons and imposing sanctions in Iraq that had resulted in the deaths of over three million children. And sprouting beneath, like malignant tumors, were paramilitary hate groups, sky-rocketing suicide rates, school-yard massacres—worse, more grotesque forms of violence than ever before.

Right around this time, *The New Yorker* ran a truly frightening article by Jerome Groopman called "The Doubting Disease: When Is Obsession a Sickness?" which, among other things, discussed the pathologization of what the author allowed might just be normal human characteristics. Preschoolers, for example, were being medicated for anxiety and depression. What drove this, one psychiatrist said, was "the free-floating anxiety that parents—often successful members of the middle and upper class—foist on their children. In the instability of today's global economy, they fear that any deviation from the norm may cripple their child's future." In the opinion of Dr. Joseph Biederman, a Harvard psychiatry professor and chief of the joint program in pediatric psychopharmacology at Massachusetts General Hospital, in fact, children were being undermedicated: "Even minor illness deserves aggressive treatment. Treat early, at the first sign, when the person is still functional." "After all," Groopman observed, "what [Biederman] and the psychologists had in common . . . was the goal of alleviating pain."[89]

I was starting to see Barbara's point. In a way, suffering was the last bastion of individuality: without the effort to find meaning through whatever portion had been parceled out to us, we became lemming-like, brain-dead clones. We wanted so badly to be different, but in our never-ending, obsessive attempt to escape suffering, we were becoming more and more the same: a kind of composite Prozac-popping, politician billionaire, spiritual guru, sports celebrity, movie star, dot-com magnate who with the same boring voice droned the same endless message: I. WANT. MORE.

I myself was no doubt a candidate for any number of antianxiety and depression medications, but the knowledge that the first thing a shrink would do was probably prescribe one of them was a chief reason I had never sought "professional" help. Delivering myself into the hands of a stranger who would be all too happy to "smooth out" my rough edges was a prospect that made my blood run cold. For all the pain they caused me, I liked my rough edges. I trusted my rough edges way more than I trusted Lilly or GlaxoSmithKline.

In fact, I'd always been perplexed by women who railed against the male-dominated power structure but thought nothing of taking birth-control pills, estrogen for menopause, and morning-after tablets. Who did they think owned the pharmaceutical companies and the ad agencies? Who, more than men out for uncommitted sex, stood to benefit from women taking birth-control pills and morning-after pills?

One day I opened the *Los Angeles Times* to find that, in spite of the risk of viruses crossing the species barrier and thereby endangering not only the life of potential organ recipients but also the general public, scientists had cloned five pigs. Aside from the unbelievably depressing attempt to reduce life to a marketable commodity, to what end, I wondered, were these people so eager to increase their life spans? What were they going to do with all that extra time: Shop? Overeat? Sue? As bloodless and grasping as the insurance companies could be, this insistence upon a "right" to be cured of every illness, a "right" to live longer than anyone else, had to be at least partly responsible for the out-of-control costs, huge premiums, and substandard health care.

And as usual, it was not the rich—not the people who were cryogenically preserving their bodies, demanding every possible experimental treatment, stridently pushing for plastic surgery, stem-cell research, and abortion on demand—who were bearing the brunt. It was the poor people, who could afford no insurance, who wanted to live, not longer lives but any kind of life at all.

23

Lay Your Sleeping Head, My Love

Agonies in bed towards morning.[90]
—Franz Kafka, Journal entry for August 15, 1913

The authorization for the oncologist, Dr. Cruz, had come through at last. In keeping with the theme that every contact with the medical profession include some element of insult, the morning of my appointment I arrived fifteen minutes early, then sat in a packed waiting room for a full hour and a half before my name was called. I'd brought along C. S. Lewis's *The Great Divorce*, and his description of hell as "the grey town" rang all too true.

Dr. Cruz, however, a dapper Hispanic man I instantly liked, turned out to be an unlikely adversary. I'd been picturing a cunning game of cat and mouse in which I asked a series of innocent questions, tripped up the good doctor, and craftily finagled him into validating my partially formed views on treatment. Instead, with the same overwrought impulsivity that had sealed my fate against trial lawyerdom, the second we shook hands I blurted, "They want me to have chemo, but I'm totally healthy! I've always had a great immune system! I don't want to have chemo!"

"Chemo can be dangerous," the doctor admitted. "It can cause leukemia; some women will even die from it. But a decrease in estrogen levels causes a corresponding decrease in recurrence rates, and the particular benefit for you is that chemo would push you into early menopause."

"But I don't want a chemically induced early menopause," I wailed. "That doesn't sound right to me one bit!"

He darted me a look, and I could almost hear him thinking, *She looks normal; she sounds normal.* . . .

"Whatever the case, you'll naturally want to have a course of hormonal therapy," he moved on suavely and began explaining the way some new wonder drug, a cousin of tamoxifen, worked: "Why, this drug whips your pituitary so hard it shuts right down!" he marveled.

"As if that could possibly be a good thing," I burst out, "as if that wouldn't necessarily create some sort of imbalance! Pretend you're not a doctor for a second. As one human being to another, doesn't it seem the tiniest bit counterproductive—wrong, even—to so cavalierly throw major systems out of whack?"

His face fell: now he knew he was dealing with a certified nut.

"Well, you have to have radiation," he pleaded. "Radiation reduces your chances of local recurrence by 20 to 30 percent."

"But will radiation improve my chances of survival?"

"Not much," he admitted. "Combined with chemotherapy in Stage 2 patients, it reduces the mortality rate by about 5 percent."

"How do they know what's attributable to chemo and what's attributable to radiation?" I inquired. "And what are the figures for Stage 1?" He didn't know; definitive studies hadn't yet been conducted.

I asked some more general questions about recurrence. Although breast cancer could resurface as long as twenty-five years later, he reported, the chances decreased markedly after five. And—exactly as I'd hoped—in the event of recurrence, the cancer usually had the same characteristics as the original tumor: the same level of aggressiveness, the same hormone factors.

I decided to lay all my cards on the table; he knew where I was heading anyway.

"What are my chances if I have no further treatment at all?" I asked.

"The five-year survival rate for Stage 1 is about 65 percent," he replied somberly.

What! A third of all Stage 1 women died within five years? Was he trying to scare me into treatment?

"How can that be?" I pressed. "Susan Love's book says 95 percent of Stage 1 patients are still alive after five years. Even with no further treatment than surgery, she posits only a 9 percent recurrence rate for Stage 1 women with tumors of 2 centimeters or less—and mine was less than 1 centimeter. At UCLA they used the same ballpark figure—9 percent."

He sighed and played with his pen and stammered around for a while, and finally he backtracked and said, "Well, taking your particular factors into consideration, you probably have about an 85 percent chance of surviving for five years—no matter what you do. But you're taking a very grave risk if you don't avail yourself of treatment. A young, healthy woman like you . . ." He shook his head in disbelief.

Solicitous and thorough, Dr. Cruz had given me a good forty minutes of his time—which I'm sure cut into his lunch hour, and for which I was deeply grateful. Still, though I'd felt a firm decision forming that morning, by the time I left his office, I'd been plunged anew into turmoil. How could I forego the benefits of chemo? How much harm, after all, could a few blasts of radiation do?

Back at home, another reign of terror began, during which I thought constantly about new lumps springing up in my breasts, tumors in my spine, cancerous bones. In my saner moments, I knew what mattered most wasn't so much the decision I made as that I based my decision on faith, not fear—but I was by no means always sane. Would prayer keep the cancer at bay? Would a good work ethic prevent the cancer from spreading to my brain? All the sages said to live in the moment, but I wasn't living in the moment at all. My mind was running manically along such lines as, *What if the cancer comes back? What if I come down with some even worse kind of illness?* Because stress compromises the immune system, I also feared that the anxiety with which I'd been burdened all my life was now going to kill me.

At the same time, I was also discovering that you can be depressed or exhausted or haunted by fear and still function; you can ignore, even embrace the discomfort. Was I still in love with the world? Yes. Part of me didn't want to be in love because leaving the world would hurt too much, but, yes, "O Lord, I love the house in which you dwell, and the place where your glory abides" (Psalm 26:8).

At Mass one morning, the Old Testament reading was from Ezra, and the priest tied in the Babylonian exile with our own exiles and transitions and dark nights that so often are undeserved and apparently for nothing. As I reflected on my own endless exile and the exile of the elderly folks gathered round in a circle for the Eucharistic prayer, I saw all over again the rightness of ordering my life around Mass. Mass was so nonspectacular, so noncataclysmic, seemingly, so not geared toward having an "experience." I wasn't interested in having an "experience"; I was interested in connecting with the rest of the world, and I was convinced that participating with people I had not personally hand-picked—the people at church being one prime example, and the people with whom I stayed sober another—was the way.

That certainly had been the way of Christ. Christ hadn't spoken of love in the abstract; he'd demonstrated it by interacting with whoever happened to be in front of him, with the individual people he'd met in the course of his day. He'd eaten, enjoyed a couple of drinks, gone to weddings and funerals; he'd come up constantly against illness, conflict, psychic bondage. During his forty days in the desert he'd seen, being fully human, that he, too, had the capacity to be tempted. He'd seen how hard it is, when you're dying of hunger and loneliness and confusion, to resist making something other than God your god.

When he returned from the desert, he hadn't tried to heal everybody. He hadn't picketed, protested, or resisted anything—except religious hypocrisy. He'd looked people in the eye with total tenderness and total clarity and told them what was wrong with them, what was blocking and weighing them down. When people came to him, he'd asked in so many words, Do you really want to be healed? Are you really willing to change—or are you just trying to get sympathy for your victimhood? He'd said, If you're so interested in being "spiritual," then feed the hungry, clothe the naked—figure out what that means. Maybe you start with clothing your own nakedness, attending to your own hunger and thirst, and then you'll be able to see other people's nakedness and hunger and thirst more clearly.

Maybe you start by shedding your cynicism and cultivating the childlike trust you had once and lost a long time ago. Really that is what Christ is about. He is about getting back to the child who is always ready to be astonished, who wears her heart on her sleeve, who is easily angered, easily hurt, and equally easily forgives—because only the childlike heart has the paradoxical strength to take on the crucifying responsibilities of adulthood.

One of the main points G. K. Chesterton makes in his spiritual classic *Orthodoxy*, in fact, is that the supposedly liberal point of view has it all wrong, that the truly liberal person is more, not less, likely to believe in miracles, the supernatural, and the power of sacrament. The rules of dogma are both stricter than the laws of science—for they make demands on the individual, requiring a response—and looser, for they are based on love and mercy. "Dogma is the guardian of mystery," noted Flannery O'Connor.[91] And ever more I saw that mystery, which the world accuses of being flabby, makes for crystal-clear decisions and a life of urgency, point, and purpose.

Dogma, for example, gave me the correct context within which to approach my marriage. That I saw marriage as a sacrament made the thought of leaving agonizing—for I was frightfully aware that I would be breaking a sacred vow—but I knew that it would also, eventually, allow me to make a decision at all and then give me the courage to follow the decision through. Dogma forbade me from hanging on to a marriage that had begun with a "defect" because I was afraid of being poor, of being alone, of being pitied, of being seen as—and of myself feeling—a failure.

To view marriage as a sacrament is to have, in a sense, the decision to stay or to go (no matter how long it might take) get "made" for you. Integrity prevents you from participating in a lie. Love dictates that for yourself and the other, depending upon the circumstances, you must stay or you must leave, no matter what the cost: financially, socially, emotionally, psychologically, and no matter what your friends or the world think. What your friends, much as you love them, think, and what the world thinks—such considerations don't even figure into any of your decisions.

In a strange way, dogma had allowed me to give up the security of my job as a lawyer and to embark on the precarious life of a writer. I had met scores of people over the past ten years, for example, who were kinder than me, more generous than me, more talented than me, smarter than me, who had told me, "I wish I could write."

The only reason I was writing and they weren't was that to me the call to write was, and had been since the day I started, sacred. To view writing as a mere career, or even as something you love and cherish very much, is different from seeing writing as a vocation, as sacred. To view the call of writing as sacred means that you *must* write. Not to write is not a matter of personal desire (though there's nothing on earth you'd rather do) or whim or practicality: not to write is a sin. You will undergo any hardship, any ignominy, any loneliness, any failure, any humiliation, any risk of being called selfish, antisocial, or insane. You believe in miracles; you believe in magic; you believe that love will reign; you believe that our hidden lives and sacrifices register; you believe that you were put on earth to write, and whether you write and what you write is a matter of life and death.

So in a quiet way, and in spite of your ongoing terrible faults and limitations, you absolutely have the courage of your convictions. And God buoys you up. Not to believe in miracles and in dogma, and then to put your trust in mere conscientiousness, mere generosity, mere talent, mere intelligence, is to work at a job you hate and to stay in a marriage that is killing you. Whereas Christ was always saying, in so many words, You are not crazy, go back to your childlike heart, your desire to have everyone around the table, your love of stories, your belief in elves and fairies and magic. Don't worry about what you're going to wear and eat and drink. Regard the lilies of the field. The Father knows what you need before you even ask for it (Matthew 6:25–34).

Do what you love, Christ says. Because what I want for you is exactly what you want for yourself.

One Saturday morning, walking up near the Fairfax District, I saw a man pushing another man down the street in a wheelchair, an Orthodox Jew, his bearded face shaded by the round brim of his black hat, headed to temple. I saw pink azaleas, calla lilies, a patch of cream-edged mint. I saw a gay couple with old kitchen items spread out on a blanket on their front lawn, having a yard sale. I saw a hollowed-out panhandler up by Melrose, the right half of the hair on her head dyed red, the left half blue. And with a kind of wrenching wonder, I thought, *What does it mean to be alive? What does it mean to be human?*

When I got home, Tim was sleeping, the black silk beauty mask he wore to shut out the light clamped over his eyes, his DayGlo orange earplugs in place, and Blanche, the ever-trusty cat, curled up beside him.

I thought of a passage from W. H. Auden:

> Lay your sleeping head, my love,
> Human on my faithless arm.[92]

Tim was so good. I loved him; I felt compassion for him. But if for no other reason than my own unworked-through wounds, I sensed we'd both begun to wonder whether we should ever have gotten married.

24

Desert Hot Springs

Whatever remedies you may use, they will only work to the
extent that he will permit. When suffering comes from God, he
alone can cure it, and he often leaves us with physical illness in
order to cure our spiritual illness. Find consolation in the
sovereign doctor of body and soul.[93]
—Brother Lawrence of the Resurrection, circa 1660

The desert is such a big Lenten theme that, as Easter approached, Tim
and I decided to spend a few days in a real desert. For years we'd been
driving out on the odd weekend to Desert Hot Springs, a kind of poor
man's Palm Springs a couple of hours east of L.A. It's always fun to
observe white people when you get them out of the city, take away
their dental care, and give them motorcycles. The town was full of
time-warp forty-dollar-a-night "spas"—Arthritis Cure! Asthma relief!
Reducing clinic! the faded signs read—where, in a cinder-block room
with mold on the windows, plastic flowers on the patio table, and a
rusty stationary bicycle in the corner, we could soak to our hearts' con-
tent in a scalding pool of piped-in mineral water.

The establishment we picked this time was called The Enchanted
Door. Tim suggested that the lady who ran it would probably like to
rename it The Undone Chores because she did all the work while the
deadbeat man of the house—husband? boyfriend? son?—sat around
all day watching TV and complaining. On our first afternoon there,

the strains of a Santana-type band that was kicking off the reopening of a rival spa down the street marred the otherwise pristine quiet. The next day, the proprietor took a break and sat out by the pool all afternoon gabbing with her girlfriend, whose boyfriend had just dumped her, and the final night, a lesbian couple rolled in and sat up half the night in their kitchen talking at full voice with the windows open, so we couldn't sleep. Other than that, the place was primo, with a very nice thermal bath and pool, comfortable lawn chairs shaded by bougainvillea and, if we stood on the bed on tiptoe, a view of the mountains.

We hiked during the day, read in the afternoon, watched the bats swoop out from the eaves at dusk, and beneath every activity ran the mental refrain that had been nagging at me for weeks: WHAT ARE YOU GOING TO DO ABOUT THE CANCER? To think of simply "letting" myself die sounded callous, but could anything be more callous than doctors who advocated potentially fatal treatments, then wanted to help you kill yourself when they didn't work? To refrain from availing myself of the wonders of modern medicine sounded to some degree crazy, but weren't human guinea pigs, falsified research, and "cures" that were worse than the disease crazy, in an even more pernicious way? Was going against medical advice passion, or was it pathology? Was it obedience, or was it insanity? I'd talked the issue over with many trusted friends and spiritual advisors, including Father Terry, and they'd all pretty much said, "The decision is between you and God."

All the self-help books said that you had to be a fighter—not a quitter! But the gung-ho American spirit that was always trying to win—the struggle against cancer, the battle against drugs, the war for democracy—had always seemed to me deeply misguided, and never more so when people tried to drag "God" into the equation. I found it impossible to believe that God intended us to safeguard the vote by dropping atomic bombs on large Japanese cities, for example, or holding drug addicts in twenty-three-hour-a-day isolation cells, or training Latin American military officers to torture, maim, and kill at the School of the Americas in Georgia. And the idea that fighting a chemical- and radiation-enhanced "battle" was going to do anything for my Stage 1, Grade 1 breast cancer but make it worse struck me now as equally and increasingly unlikely.

The one place I'd gotten on board with Sontag's *Illness as Metaphor*, in fact, was with her description of the "military flavor" of cancer treatments:

> The controlling metaphors in descriptions of cancer are . . . drawn not from economics but from the language of warfare: every physician and every attentive patient is familiar with, if perhaps inured to, this medical terminology. Thus, cancer cells do not simply multiply; they are "invasive." . . . Cancer cells "colonize" from the original tumor to far sites in the body. . . .
>
> Treatment also has a military flavor. Radiotherapy uses the metaphors of aerial warfare; patients are "bombarded" with toxic rays. And chemotherapy is chemical warfare, using poisons. . . . Treatment aims to "kill" cancer cells (without, it is hoped, killing the patient). Unpleasant side effects of treatment are advertised, indeed overadvertised. ("The agony of chemotherapy" is a standard phrase.) It is impossible to avoid damaging or destroying healthy cells (indeed, some methods used to treat cancer can cause cancer), but it is thought that nearly any damage to the body is justified if it saves the patient's life. Often, of course, it doesn't work. (As in, "We had to destroy Ben Suc in order to save it.") There is everything but the body count.[94]

Where I didn't get on board with Sontag was that she seemed less outraged at war than simply outraged. She was irritated by doctors who were overly optimistic about cancer, and she was irritated by doctors who were overly pessimistic about cancer.[95] She was irritated that disease is equated with death (not, it must be said, an entirely moronic or far-fetched equation), irritated that to use cancer as a metaphor "amounts to saying, first of all, that the event or situation is irredeemably wicked."[96] She was irritated that to describe a phenomenon as a cancer is an "incitement to violence,"[97] irritated that to equate cancer with evil is "implicitly genocidal,"[98] and irritated that the cultural view of cancer is "invariably an encouragement to simplify what is complex and an invitation to self-righteousness if not fanaticism."[99]

Which all struck me as wildly melodramatic: I was no supporter of the cultural view of cancer (or the cultural view of much of anything), but it was hardly as if heads of state were ordering cancer patients to be lined up and shot. The insult of cancer, to Sontag, was not to the sick or suffering of the whole world; the insult was to her, and no amount of the high dudgeon that ensued could mask the flimsiness of her argument or the inconsistency of her stance.

Because, interestingly, while deploring the military metaphor, in the end Sontag also availed herself of the metaphor. While railing against the inhuman treatments, she also actively sought out and submitted to the most inhuman treatments available. The idea for the book came after she had already suffered a radical mastectomy for her own breast cancer.[100] Later she would undergo an "extreme thirty-month course of chemotherapy with massive doses of certain drugs that had not yet received FDA approval."[101] "Chemotherapy was agony. There were also follow-up and exploratory operations."[102] She counseled her friends to undergo painful, agonizing surgery as well.[103] Her actions seemed to spring from, and to give rise to, further anger. "[F]ighting cancer gave Sontag a sense of release," noted one biographer.[104] "When she typed the words 'death,' 'agony,' 'cancer,' she laughed and said 'I've won.' She wrote [*Illness as Metaphor*] in a kind of controlled rage."[105]

Sontag professed to abhor violence, in other words, and yet she availed herself of violence. She professed to decry war, and yet her whole life was geared toward fighting—and winning. That is the problem when you refuse to admit of the spiritual and the mystical. You can only complain. You have no possible response to life but archness, irony, distaste, distance, dismissal. You can see only that something is wrong, but you can't see in what way it's wrong, or the extent and substance of the error, or that you yourself contribute to what is wrong, or that there's any hope or any solution. You can only sneer at both sides, then reluctantly join one of them. You can only submit yourself to agonizing treatments, make a career out of refusing to suffer "fools" gladly, and wait for science to come up with a cure based on the body's natural defenses and the "immunodefensive system"[106]—as if the body operated independently of the heart, the conscience, the soul.

But until then (and don't hold your breath waiting), you have nothing. You have a world in which everything and everybody is wrong but you. You have a world that you see as absurd and yet in which you feel constantly "forced" to go along with what is absurd; to compromise your integrity, intellectual and otherwise, because you have no truth, no compass, no North Star.

And to cover up for your lack of a North Star, you bluster. "Who are the writers you light candles to?" interviewer Chris Lydon once asked Sontag. "I don't light candles to anyone," she replied testily. "I don't light candles to writers. I *am* a writer."[107]

To cover up the fact that you have no North Star, you issue fiats. "[P]eople had to be shown that they were not responsible for causing their illnesses," Sontag decreed. People were "obligated to resist [their illnesses] by seeking out the best possible treatment."[108]

But obligated by whom or by what? Without insurance, Sontag had paid for her own "best possible" treatment by appealing to the writers organization PEN. When PEN turned her down, a friend came up with the $150,000.[109] Which was lovely, but weren't those who really had a right to be pissed the zillions of people around the world, with or without breast cancer, who didn't have access to a hundred dollars, never mind 150 grand?

But nothing struck me as more cockamamie than her insistence that we should adopt a new, politically correct way (her way) of speaking and thinking about cancer. Don't allude to the fact that people croak from cancer right and left, was her idea: that might cause the cancer-afflicted to fall into despair and prevent them from seeking treatment. Huh? Wouldn't knowing you could die *encourage* you to seek treatment? Plus, that cancer kills is news? Plus, people do what they want to do. Plus, political correctness is never about actually helping the people it purports to protect; it's about the person who insists on political correctness being in control.

Would forbidding the use of the phrase "falling-down drunk" get even one falling-down drunk sober? Would refraining from describing AIDS as a scourge make AIDS one whit less of a lacerating, blood-dripping scourge? Would outlawing the words *halt, lame, blind, crippled,* and *leper* help the lame, blind, crippled, and leprous to feel one whit more welcome, more accepted, more loved? No. Other people do that. We help one another feel welcome and loved. Personally, calling cancer a scourge, a plague, a pestilence helped me to be *more* compassionate toward the person afflicted with it, not less.

As for my own cancer, my dilemma, as I saw it, was this: I had a mystical duty to be a good steward of my body, and I had a (possible) civic duty to go along with the "law" of prevailing medical advice.

As a Catholic, however, I was allowed—even called—to break immoral laws:

"The strict conditions for *legitimate defense by military force* require rigorous consideration. The gravity of such a decision makes it subject to rigorous conditions of moral legitimacy. . . . The evaluation of these conditions [of the 'just war' doctrine] for moral legitimacy belongs to the prudential judgment of those who have responsibility for the common good" [*Catechism of the Catholic Church*, 2309].

"If rulers were to enact unjust laws or take measures contrary to the moral order such arrangements would not be binding in conscience" [*Catechism*, 1903].

"Blind obedience [to immoral laws] does not suffice to excuse those who carry them out" [*Catechism*, 2313].

And from a 2003 pastoral letter from the Bishop of the Diocese of Canton, Ohio: "When a moral conflict arises between Church teaching and secular morality, when contradictory moral demands are made upon a Catholic's conscience, he or she 'must obey God rather than man' (Acts 5:29)."[110]

I was by no means antimedicine. If I'd had an infection, I would have had no trouble taking penicillin. I'd been all for the lumpectomy. Broken leg, car crash, God forbid, I'd be at the ER in a trice. But penicillin and/or surgery don't make your hair and fingernails fall out, give you secondary cancers, and possibly kill you. In fact, I'd even looked up the way penicillin works, which is basically by osmosis, and you don't need twelve years of medical school to see that osmosis is a whole different deal than poisoning or burning.

I wasn't angling for a miraculous healing or cure. I wasn't particularly drawn to holistic or alternative treatments any more than I was to chemo and radiation. I just wanted to keep doing what I was doing, which, problems notwithstanding, was living as fully as I could. I just didn't want to live a lie. I just didn't want to feel forced into a course of action I found absurd.

I knew that for a layperson to do a smattering of online research and purport to dispense her own medical advice was in one sense laughable. I knew that to link cancer treatments with war was a stretch. But nonviolence is not only, or even primarily, a stance toward war. Nonviolence is a stance toward life.

Nonviolence isn't practical—this objection was always raised. In fact, nonviolence is practical, and I knew because I had seen the results from practicing it, however imperfectly, in my own life. I had seen the results when I made my goal in a conflict not to win an advantage but to resolve the conflict. I had seen the results of copping to my hatreds, jealousies, resentments; taking them to the Sacrament of Reconciliation; making amends, as best I could, to the people I'd hurt; and letting the other person off the hook for the hurt he or she had done to me.

But most of all, I had seen the counterintuitive, utterly unlikely, and yet graphic results of "nonviolence" with respect to treating the vicious, often fatal disease of alcoholism.

Temperance crusader Carrie Nation had battered down saloon doors with hatchets; the fellowship I'd found worked by accepting the alcoholic as he or she was and inviting that person to a higher place. Psychiatry wanted to treat alcoholism with pills, chemicals, clinicians, and therapies; the way I'd found was simple, personal, free, and consisted at its core of one wounded alcoholic talking to another. Science had established multimillion-dollar research centers to study the alcoholic's nervous system and brain circuitry; the way I'd found involved looking into and purifying my heart.

And the way I'd found had worked. It had worked where no amount of intelligence backed by willpower had worked. It had worked when no amount of the violence of shame, reproach, and self-flagellation had worked. Science had sent rockets to the moon, but it had not found a way to treat my alcoholism. Science went so far, but science could not explain why or how I, a hopeless, falling-down drunk, had not had a drink for thirteen years.

Of course, to say that nonviolence is practical does not derogate the fact that people also may very well kill you, Christ being the prime example. Nonviolence may not work in the short run, but it always works in the long run. Violence inevitably, boringly, predictably, generates more violence. Whereas the nonviolent love of Christ creates ripples that go out in all directions and that, just as inevitably, generate more peace, more nonviolent love. In fact, nonviolence "works" in the short run, too, even if they do kill you, because the highest sense of "to work" in this case means that you're freed up to operate from the highest love and the highest joy. You, yourself, are set free from hatred and violence and guilt.

Sontag was right to see the link between guilt and the lack of self-love that might prevent a person from seeking treatment. She was right to observe that we often feel guilty for things we didn't do, or because we tend to view our afflictions as punishment, even if no logical or visible connection exists. But guilt isn't relieved by censorship. Guilt isn't relieved by decreeing that people should think or talk a certain way. Guilt isn't relieved by irritation, anger, or playing the *grande dame*.

Guilt is relieved by repentance and mercy. Getting sober had for me been a Prodigal-Daughter experience of being welcomed back to the human table. The experience had transformed me. I firmly believed that spiritual laws had to hold true across the board, and if I'd been a scientist, I would have devoted my entire life to researching how all of matter, both human and nonhuman, lives and moves and has its being in a way that is completely conversant with the Gospels.

The Gospels tell us that the highest thing is not health. The highest thing is not even life. The highest thing is love. And in order to love ourselves, we have to take account of our wounds, our temperaments, our limitations. Given my own particular emotional baggage and sense of bodily integrity, I'm not sure I would not rather have died than have my breast amputated. I'm not sure I would not rather have died than deliver my body into the hands of doctors who were on such a radically different wavelength than mine.

You can argue with that stance, you can find fault with that stance, but the legitimacy of that stance was not for anyone else to say. If I could not undertake the recommended treatment without feeling that I was doing violence to myself, then for me—not necessarily for anyone else, but for me—the toward-God action was to go against medical advice.

One set of facts my fevered brain circled back to again and again: in spite of all the brouhaha over the supposed advance in treatments, the survival rate for breast cancer had not appreciably improved in the last thirty years. In spite of the walkathons and public health bulletins, the Revlon Breast Center with its teak paneling and tasteful wig boutique, and the omniscient Dr. Love, the fact remained that nobody knew what caused breast cancer, nobody could predict what course breast cancer would run, and nobody knew how to cure breast cancer. Exactly as with alcoholism, the medical community attacked as best they could from the outside and hoped for the best.

But I had never been much drawn, convinced, or transformed by what happened on the outside. The law imposed itself from the outside; the spirit worked its mystery from the inside. Capitalism was based on competition, aggression, and the notion of scarcity; the kingdom of God was based on the certainty of overflowing abundance. The medical system was geared toward living as long as you possibly could; mysticism said the goal was to live life fully, even if you died young. The world said to hedge your bets; Christ had bet every last thing he had on the Father. As followers of Christ we were called to accept our fragile selves, love our enemies, and forgive the murderer. As with our "battles" against drugs, cancer, and terrorism, instead we poisoned, amputated, incarcerated, shunned, rejected, attacked, discarded, burned, and killed.

I knew from my experience with legal research that I'd eventually reach a point with my exploration of breast cancer when I'd know that

I'd taken in as much information as I needed to, that I was on the verge of forming a coherent, fleshed-out picture, that to stop was safe.

Our last morning in the desert I woke before dawn, crept out to the pool, watched the sky lighten from violet to cobalt to pink-stippled blue. By the time the sun came over the mountains in a blaze of gold, I thought, *I've almost reached that point now.*

25

No Turning Back

It's only a short time since I really understood what the cross is. It is simultaneously miraculous and horrifying. Miraculous, because it gives us life, horrifying because if we do not bring about our own crucifixion, we have no access to life. This is the great and blessed mystery for those who are persecuted.[111]
—*Light upon the Scaffold: Prison Letters of Jacques Fesch*

Palm Sunday, the Sunday before Easter, commemorates Christ's triumphal entry into Jerusalem, a week before the very crowd that welcomed him would turn and cry for his crucifixion. That the Son of Man had come into his glory not on a white steed but a donkey, not with an armed retinue but with a ragtag band of disciples, one of whom would soon betray him, and not with a chorus of celestial trumpet blasts but with a boisterous crowd paving his way with humble palm fronds, was just the kind of counterintuitive drama that stirred my heart.

If you have followed along during Lent and kept even a measly kind of fast and prayer, then the events of Holy Week—the slow buildup, the passion play of the Crucifixion and Resurrection that begins on Palm Sunday—have an almost unendurable emotional force. Back in L.A. I'd decided to celebrate by attending morning Mass on Palm Sunday at a South-L.A. church that was renowned for its gospel choir.

As I headed down Crenshaw—the main thoroughfare from Koreatown to South L.A.—I wished for the thousandth time that Tim were beside me, but I'd converted alone, for the most part I went to Mass alone, and no one was more aware than I that if I really wanted to call myself a follower of Christ, maybe I could be a little kinder to and more tolerant of my husband. Still, the pang went deep. That I could not share my love for Christ meant that I could not share the ground of my life. And that I could not share the ground of my life meant that the decision I was about to make had to be made apart—and very far away—from the person closest to me.

I'd never been to this particular parish before, but the scene in the parking lot alone told me that I was in for half religious service/half high theater: women dolled up in gold mules and glittery dresses, little girls with cornrows intricately dressed in barrettes, a man sporting an iridescent turquoise suit. I threaded through the throng, made my way inside, and squeezed into a pew near the back. A woman in an emerald-green turban cased the aisles, handing out complimentary fans embossed with the name of a local funeral home. Flamboyantly arrayed families paraded and preened. Folks shouted greetings, high-fived, beamed, and flashed their jewelry, teeth, eyes.

Then Mass began. Dashiki-clad drumbeaters led the processional; the lectors climbed a set of stairs to the pulpit and read as if their lungs were being torn from their chests; the priest trembled and railed; and the choir, dressed to the nines, interposed their showboating, amplified histrionics at every turn. This was so not what I'd expected! I'd pictured the Dixie Hummingbirds, not *Star Search*; a cappella harmonies, not booming mikes! I felt small, bland, tense, and comically, hopelessly white against the backdrop of rolling organs and soaring trills, shouting and clapping, the waving of paper fans.

Still, I was among people without having to speak to them—one of the many reasons I had always loved Mass. Besides, who would deny Christ, on the eve of his Passion, such pageantry, such parrot hues? How to fathom the inclusiveness of a Savior who, no matter our background, history, culture, demographic, gender, or genealogy, acknowledged our desperate hunger to belong? How to comprehend the strangeness of a Church that took so many shapes, the Mansion in which there were so many rooms, from Gothic cathedrals to monastic cells to this amplified, peacock-feather of a sanctuary in South L.A.? How grateful I was to be held to its capacious bosom! How humbled I was by a Savior who did not pander or reward or protect from suffering but, out of love, suffered with us.

The last of the three readings at Sunday Mass is always from one of the four Gospels. But on Palm Sunday the congregation takes a part, too, and along with the priest and various others (the Narrator, Peter, Pilate), together we read the entire pages-long Passion story, this year from the book of Mark:

> Then the high priest stood up before them and asked Jesus, "Have you no answer? What is it that they testify against you?" But he was silent and did not answer. Again the high priest asked him, "Are you the Messiah, the Son of the Blessed One?" Jesus said, "I am; and 'you will see the Son of Man seated at the right hand of the Power,' and 'coming with the clouds of heaven.'"
>
> Then the high priest tore his clothes and said, "Why do we still need witnesses? You have heard his blasphemy! What is your decision?" All of them condemned him as deserving death (Mark 14:60–64). . . .
>
> Pilate asked him, "Are you the King of the Jews?" He answered him, "You say so." Then the chief priests accused him of many things. Pilate asked him again, "Have you no answer? See how many charges they bring against you." But Jesus made no further reply, so that Pilate was amazed (Mark 15:2–5).

So that Pilate was amazed.

I was amazed as well. I was amazed at the purity of heart required to voluntarily take the last place and let someone else take the first. I was amazed, endlessly, about the paradoxical "triumph" of love over failure, exile, and death.

I thought of how Christ had gone not against the system but beyond it.

I thought of the martyrs who had gone to their deaths singing.

I thought how, of all the people who had helped me over the past few months, the one most deeply enshrined in my memory was not a professional, a volunteer, a "survivor," or even a friend, but a fellow sufferer: the lady at UCLA with the ash-blonde wig.

That was "how things worked": not through even the highest forms of philosophy, medicine, law, politics, or technology; not by progress, efficiency, or statistics, but by the inexplicable, sublime largeness of heart that wished another well when—for no good, logical, fair reason—you were in agony yourself. The largeness of heart of Christ on the cross, assuring the repentant thief beside him: "Truly I tell you, today you will be with me in Paradise" (Luke 23:43). The largeness of heart of the boy on my left, who shyly offered me his small, warm hand as we stood for the Lord's Prayer.

Blessed are the poor in spirit: the out-of-step, the unhappy in marriage, the mistake makers, the frightened, the sick, the uncertain, the lonely, the yearning, the oppressed. Because only the poor in spirit know the incalculable value, the infinite preciousness, of a fellow human hand.

I didn't expect the people who treated my cancer to be my best friends; what I objected to was the lie, the sin of omission. The doctors who failed to say, Cancer is a mystery to us. We have no cure. We can maybe stave it off with chemicals and burning that may or may not work and that may or may not cause more suffering than you would have undergone anyway. The health-care system that was an extension of the same massive PR program-lie of the "American way," a country that claimed to be based on peace but that was really based on the wholesale murder of war. A country that claimed to be for the people but was really for the rich people. A country that claimed to be based on God but was really based on money. The culture that claimed we can have it all: a fat bank account, eternal youth, sanitized, hygienic perfection. Where was the honesty? Where was the humility? Where was the Person who would cherish our souls?

We heard a testosterone-fueled version of "There Is a Balm in Gilead." We were bombarded with the lyrics: "Je-sus all RIGHT (beat), Je-sus all RIGHT (beat), Je-sus all right (beat, beat), WITH me."

But the song that really got to me went,

> I've decided to follow Jesus,
> I've decided to follow Jesus,
> I've decided to follow Jesus,
> No turnin' back.
> No turnin' back.[112]

A thousand feet stamped. Five hundred palm fronds rattled. The smell of Jheri Curl wafted across the pews. That was when I finally lost it, covered my face with my hands, and wept. In a sanctuary full of singing, swaying strangers, I had made my decision. I was done. I wasn't going to have any more treatment.

26

Good-bye to All That

The Catholic writer, in so far as he has the mind of the Church, will feel life from the standpoint of the central Christian mystery: that it has for all its horror, been found by God to be worth dying for.[113]
—Flannery O'Connor

One afternoon a month or so later, for the last time I undressed, put on a johnny, and stood staring out a ninth-story window of the Mercy General Medical Building at the smog-shrouded San Gabriel mountains. Staggers came in, shook my hand, and began probing my breast.

"All finished with chemo?" he asked jovially.

"Oh, I'm not doing chemo."

His smile faded.

"So you're in the middle of radiation?"

"No, I'm not doing radiation, either," I told him. "I'm not doing anything."

His fingers stopped.

"Well, it's your decision," he said stiffly. "Obviously a very unwise decision."

"Around the stitches is still a little sore," I offered quickly, hoping he wouldn't elaborate. "That's why I came in."

He didn't really respond, just felt around some more and said, "Hmm, there's some thickening."

"Everything's all right, though?" I asked.

"Yes," he said, and let my johnny fall back into place.

"So why did you decide to do nothing?" he asked as he was writing in my chart.

I wanted to say, Because life is a mystery that neither of us understands, because we are two human beings trapped in a system that makes it impossible for us to show compassion for one another, because if my time is going to be cut short, I want to spend the least amount of the remaining time possible in a doctor's office.

Instead, I said, "I guess a variety of factors: spiritual, religious, philosophical."

"You can be spiritual and still have medical treatment," he snapped.

"Yes, I know," I said, "but after a lot of research"—("and prayer," I was going to add, but I couldn't quite bring myself to utter the word in that sterile, sanitary room)—"I came to the conclusion that for me, at this stage of the game anyway, those invasive treatments would do more harm than good."

"Invasive!" he scoffed. "Chemo, maybe, but radiation and tamoxifen aren't invasive at all!"

"But it's not your body!" I said. "I took birth control pills in my twenties, and I know how they made me feel, and I don't want to tamper with my hormone system again. And there are side effects, and radiation doesn't increase your chances of survival one bit." My words came out in a tangled rush, the plea of a disobedient child or of a criminal for mercy.

"I can't believe that radiation doesn't increase your chances of surviving," he snorted.

"It's true!" I said. "Even the oncologist basically admitted as much."

"I don't believe it," he repeated stubbornly. "Radiation vastly decreases the risk of local recurrence."

"Yeah, weird isn't it?" I commiserated. "But that's what they've found. Just as many women eventually die anyway."

"Well, if you'll allow me to," he sniffed, "I'd like you to come in six months from now so I can examine your breasts. And you should have a mammogram in January."

"Okay, thank you," I said. He had done the best he could, after all, and I suddenly felt sorry for him.

"Thank you very much for your help!" I called again, but the door had already closed.

I got dressed, took the elevator down to the lobby, and as I had that long-ago day in January, stopped in at the chapel. Same oyster-shell font, same cheesy piped-in music, same corporate fabric-upholstered chairs, same me, minus a small chunk of my left breast—and Christ ever alive, ever new.

I knelt and reflected that I could hardly believe the hidden, steadfast way I'd been led over the course of the past few months: every article, book, conversation, and especially, person, placed in my path at the exact moment needed to impart maximum balance and sanity. Out of the days when the shadow of death had not been out of my mind for more than five seconds at a stretch and the nights when I obsessively turned over in my mind the cold statistics and mortality rates, molecule by molecule a resolve had been built. Even the delays and snafus, I saw now, had served a purpose, giving me all the time I needed to come to a decision that felt right. Thank you, my Lord. . . . Thank you. . . . Thank you. . . .

And then I got up, dipped my fingers in holy water, crossed myself, and walked through the lobby and out the front door of Mercy General, thinking, *Nobody's going to stop me; nobody's going to strap me down; nobody's going to run toxic chemicals into my veins.* Heading for my car, I started up the flower-lined path that runs between the clinic and the main hospital, passing the friendly beds of myrtle, the hopeful impatiens, faster and faster, my heart beating in time to the refrain, "I'm free I'm free, I'm FREEEEE!!!"

By the time I got to the top of the hill, I was sprinting.

I like to think that cancer showed me the strength of my faith, but 91 percent or 85 percent or even 65 percent are pretty good odds, and another possibility is that I have no faith at all. Was refusing to avail myself of putatively beneficial medical treatment the sign of some sinister neurosis? Do I have a subconscious death wish? Even I can't know my true motives, but then again, maybe that's part of the risk of faith; maybe stumbling blindly forward in spite of one's ignorance *is* faith.

I am grateful for modern surgery, and I know that if my cancer had been even slightly more advanced, I might well have made—and, should the cancer recur, might well make in the future—a different decision. I know, too, that my dilemma was a luxury that millions of women without access to top-notch medical care will never have. I know that for another woman, treatment would have been the victory, the answered prayer. Someone else would have discovered different statistics or interpreted the ones I discovered in a different way. Someone else would have come—rightly—to a different decision.

But if I'd had treatment, the reason would have been because I was thinking, *It might permanently screw me up, and it'll hurt like hell, and I don't really believe it works, and the people who administer it don't give a hoot about me, but I'm so afraid of dying I'm going to do those things anyway.* To submit myself to treatment, under the circumstances, would have meant going along with someone else's idea of life, when my own idea was radically different.

Refusing treatment was what my intuition and heart told me to do, but what, left to my own devices, I would never have had the courage to do. And in spite of the nights when I still jolt awake in a cold sweat, the terror I still feel at the thought of finding another lump, the grief that kicks me in the gut every time I hear that yet another woman's life has been cut short by breast cancer, to have followed my heart is still worth more to me than any time I could have "bought" with chemo or radiation. I would have jolted awake and felt terrified and grieved, in any case. I might die of cancer, but I'm going to die, someday, anyway.

The day I sat in the radiology room at Mercy General pondering Rilke's question—"Must I write?"—seems a lifetime ago. In a way, I had already answered yes, but I hadn't yet known the full dimensions of the yes. I had not understood that a yes of that magnitude contains many noes. I could not know that the country to which I passed over that day would turn out to be not so much the country of the ill as the country of the fully committed.

Outwardly, my life is much the same as it was before the diagnosis. I spend my days at my desk. I write, send out manuscripts, and correspond with readers, as I have for years. I sit quietly in the morning with my breviary; I take a walk in the afternoon; I examine my conscience at night. At the center, as always, is the Eucharist.

The difference is that the beauty of this simple, struggling existence is all the more piercing to me now because the scars hidden beneath my shirt—the line carved by the scalpel, the gash where the lymph node came out—only remind me that my time on earth may be shorter than I'd hoped, that we are more vulnerable than we can ever imagine, that the angel of God has hands of fire and that none of us emerges unsinged. Now I know that what makes us human is not our strengths, our triumphs, the battles we win, but our defects and frailties—and that we are loved and can in turn love others, not in spite of, but because of, them.

For to love is to die, and to die—for Christ, for beauty—is to have life eternal. Hitler perished in his bunker; Anne Frank lives on. James

Earl Ray molders; Martin Luther King Jr. is perpetually reborn. The inventor of the atom bomb is already a footnote, but every December 25th the world stops to remember the coming of a baby.

Maybe my mission in Koreatown was not, after all, to hear a new message but to be stripped down so that I could learn the only message there is, in the last way I would have chosen myself. Because now I know that where I live or whether my cancer comes back doesn't really matter. Now I know that what matters is not whether I suffer but that I offer my suffering to the world.

Now I know that the worst thing is not, after all, death. The worst thing would be dying without having hungered to know, with every last breath, for what and for whom I'd lived.

Epilogue

God is at home. We are in the far country.[114]
—Meister Eckhart, thirteenth-century German theologian
and mystic

Fifteen years later, *Dr. Susan Love's Breast Book*, periodically updated, still sells briskly. Ralph W. Moss and Samuel Epstein are still railing against the cancer establishment. Women are still dying of breast cancer.

But the opinions of the medical community have changed—are changing—will change again.

As of 2002, the American Medical Association, which for years had been urging hormone replacement therapy (HRT) upon menopausal women, for example, did an about-face, admitted that the risks of estrogen—breast cancer, heart attacks, strokes—outweighed the benefits and issued a new recommendation that women should take the lowest feasible dose of HRT for the shortest possible amount of time.[115]

Similarly, after years of recommending that, starting at age forty, women have annual mammograms, in early 2010 the US Preventive Services Task Force suddenly announced, Don't have mammograms every year. Unless you have a family history of breast cancer, don't start until you're fifty, and then only biennially. Don't bother with self-exams—they don't save lives. [116]

Perhaps most noteworthy, from the perspective of this book, is that while all along doctors had been recommending chemo and radiation to every woman with breast cancer, regardless of the stage or grade of the disease, the Task Force also admitted that "1% to 10% of cancers found through mammograms turn out to be essentially harmless, because *they will never prove life-threatening*" [emphasis mine].[117]

In other words, at long last, doctors are admitting that they've been overtreating breast cancer. Finally the medical establishment is acknowledging that tens of thousands of women have been cavalierly exposed to the severe side effects of chemo and radiation who neither needed, nor benefited from, such treatments. And, of course, in a way, chemo and radiation are the least of the horror. Every so often I think of the day I sat in the oncologist's office and he gave me my "choice": a lumpectomy with radiation—or a mastectomy without.

I offer this information not to prove that I was "right"—I was graced; I was extraordinarily lucky—but to say that while medical opinions change, the inward look never changes, never becomes outdated, ever brings forth fresh, unexpected fruit.

The point is not to excoriate the medical profession but, trapped as its members are in a system the goal of which is not healing, but profit, to mourn for them, too. The point is not to promote one avenue of treatment, thinking, or action over another but to foster compassion for the sick and suffering throughout the world, many of whom are panic stricken, in pain, illiterate, poor, and alone. The point is that, maybe more than we know, the potential for healing lies within ourselves. Not necessarily physical healing, but the spiritual healing by which we learn that the real tragedy is to die with our truest song unsung—to die without recognizing that our suffering has meaning.

When we're suffering, we don't feel it has meaning; we don't much care whether it has meaning. The helpers don't help; the darkness often doesn't lift. To choose to believe that the darkness will give way to light anyway—somehow, sometime—is a fearsome challenge, an almost unbearable responsibility.

The responsibility is to live fully now, to come awake no matter what our physical or emotional condition might be: "Therefore, keep awake—for you do not know when the master of the house will come" (Mark 13:35), and that is both an invitation and an admonition. To question how we spend our time and money; to examine our relationships to food, people, work, our bodies; to acknowledge our complicity in the suffering of the world is a daunting task. Because if we truly want to come awake, chances are that we are going to have to let go of some things. We are going to have to change. We are going to have to suffer in ways we probably would not have chosen for ourselves.

So I'm not glad I got cancer. I mourn the fact that anyone else has ever had to deal with or has died from cancer. I do not view my cancer as a lesson or a blessing or a gift; I view my cancer as a mystery. That's one reason I have never had a desire to run a Cancer Survivor 10k or carry a Cancer Survivor Mylar balloon or wear a Cancer Survivor pink ribbon. I have a desire to live every moment to the hilt. I have a desire to seek God's will. I have a desire to learn how to lay down my life for my friends.

One major event occurred in the wake of the year I've described here: my marriage crumbled. Cancer brought to a crisis many warring impulses: the impulse to put others first versus the necessity of putting myself first (for you can only love others as well and as fully as you love yourself); the impulse toward financial security versus the knowledge that true security lies in God; the impulse to observe that some people are capable of having both a vocation as a writer and a relationship versus the realization that I may not be one of them. We both gave everything we had, but perhaps no marriage ever truly survives a death at the beginning, and therefore forever at the center, of it.

In ending my marriage, I was guided by none other than Dante's Beatrice:

> Beatrice . . . gives us a hint of one way to test the validity of . . . a breaking of commitment. Be sure, she says, that the new way of life which you choose demands more of you than the old, in the proportion of six to four. . . . In other words, the breaking of a vow must be at its roots a sacrifice (a making holy), a movement toward wholeness, not an escape.[118]

That the new life has demanded more than the old has certainly proved to be the case. My responsibilities have grown, not lessened. I've been invited to give more, not to keep more.

Letting go of one thing, and one person, that were dear to me, moreover (and yes, we're still friends!), has led to letting go of many others. Without the security of a husband, I've been called to deepen my prayer life and to lean more on my friends. I eventually resigned from the State Bar of California (a door I'd always kept ajar "just in case"), realizing that no matter how badly I need money, I never again wanted to devote myself to work about which I was morally ambivalent.

In 2010, I gave notice on my apartment—the apartment in which I became a writer and a Catholic; the apartment in which I learned I had cancer—gave away or sold many of my belongings, and set out for a six-month sabbatical in which to explore in greater depth many of the issues set forth in this book: the tension between solitude and community; the link between mind, body, and spirit; the notions of responsibility, mercy, and forgiveness.

I've learned this much: no matter how long or how short our time, no matter how seemingly senseless our pain, our struggles have incalculable significance and worth. My own struggles continue. I can be testy, and I also sometimes surprise myself with my patience. I still tend to drive myself too hard, but I'm also a little more likely to give myself and everyone else a break. I worry where my next buck will come from, but recently I also had the great honor of sitting at the bedside of a dying friend.

Still, I read, puzzle, ponder. Still, I'm obsessed with how things work. Still, I wake in the night and ask, What does it mean to be human?

And last spring, I had my first mammogram in years.

It came back "Normal."

Endnotes

1. Octavio Paz, "The Day of the Dead" in *The Labyrinth of Solitude and Other Writings* (New York: Grove Press, 1994), 57.

2. Rainer Maria Rilke, *Letters to a Young Poet*, trans. M. D. Herter Norton (New York: W. W. Norton & Company, 1934), 16.

3. St. John of the Cross, Saying 100 from "The Sayings of Light and Love," *The Collected Works of St. John of the Cross*, trans. Kieran Kavanaugh, OCD (Washington, D.C.: Institute of Carmelite Studies, 1991), 92.

4. Blaise Pascal, "The Fundamentals of the Christian Religion" in *Thoughts* (New York: P. F. Collier & Son, 1910), 187.

5. Robert Thomsen, *Bill W: The Absorbing and Deeply Moving Life Story of Bill Wilson, Co-Founder of Alcoholics Anonymous* (Center City, MN: Hazelden Foundation, 1999), 325.

6. E. F. Schumacher, *Small Is Beautiful: Economics as if People Mattered* (New York, Harper & Row, 1973), 100.

7. Clarence Jordan, *Essential Writings* (Modern Spiritual Master Series) (Maryknoll, NY: Orbis Books, 2003), 153.

8. Gerard Manley Hopkins, *Poems and Prose*, ed. W. Gardner (New York: Penguin Books, 1985), 30.

9. "The Lunatic in the Pew: Confessions of a Natural-born Catholic" http://bcm.bc.edu/issues/summer_2003/ft_natural.html.

10. Tennessee Williams, *The Night of the Iguana* (New York: Dramatists Play Service, 1998), 24.

11. Quay Brothers, "Through a Glass Darkly: Interview with the Quay Brothers," conducted by André Habib for *Senses of Cinema*, October, 2001, http://sensesofcinema.com/2002/feature-articles/quay/.

12. G. K. Chesterton, *What's Wrong With the World* (London: Catholic Way Publishing, 2013), 24.

13. Flannery O'Connor, letter to "A.", August 9, 1955, in *The Habit of Being: Letters of Flannery O'Connor* (New York: Farrar, Straus and Giroux, 1988), 93.

14. Susan M. Love, MD, with Karen Lindsey, *Dr. Susan Love's Breast Book* (New York: Perseus Books, 1995), 207–8.

15. Ibid., 203.

16. Ibid., 193.

17. C. G. Jung, *The Archetypes and the Collective Unconscious* (New York: The Bollingen Foundation, 1959), 116.

18. Ron Rolheiser, OMI, "Gethsemane—The Place of Moral Loneliness," February 20, 2005, http://ronrolheiser.com/gethsemane-the-place-of-moral-loneliness/#.VGojiPkgqm4.

19. Aleksandr Solzhenitsyn, *Cancer Ward* (New York: Noonday Press, 1968), 263.

20. Isaiah 38:14.

21. Psalm 118:12.

22. Psalm 43:5.

23. The Boston Women's Health Collective, *Our Bodies, Ourselves for the New Century* (New York: Simon and Schuster, 1998), 630.

24. The Boston Women's Health Collective, *The New Our Bodies, Ourselves* (New York: Simon and Schuster, 1998), 624–5.

25. Robert A. Johnson, *Owning Your Own Shadow: Understanding the Dark Side of the Psyche* (New York: HarperCollins, 1991), 28–29.

26. Jean-Pierre de Caussade, *Abandonment to Divine Providence*, trans. John Beevers (New York: Image, 1975), 39, 53.

27. *The Cloud of Unknowing*, trans. Clifton Wolters (Baltimore: Penguin, 1961), 76.

28. Susan M. Love, MD, with Karen Lindsey, *Dr. Susan Love's Breast Book.* (New York: Perseus Books, 1995), 265.

29. Ibid., 267.

30. Franz Kafka, from a letter to Minze Eisner, winter 1922–23, in *Letters to Friends, Family, and Editors*, trans. Richard and Clara Winston (Berlin: Schocken Books, 1977), 368.

31. Susan M. Love, MD, with Karen Lindsey, *Dr. Susan Love's Breast Book.* (New York: Perseus Books, 1995), 379–80.

32. Richard Rohr, "Living on the Edge," *Radical Grace* 19, no. 2 (November 6, 2008), The Center for Action and Contemplation.

33. Albert Camus, *Notebooks 1951–1959* (Chicago: Ivan R. Dee, 2008), 188.

34. Flannery O'Connor, *Mystery and Manners: Occasional Prose* (New York: Farrar, Straus and Giroux, 1961), 189.

35. Bernie Siegel, MD, *Peace, Love, and Healing* (New York: William Morrow, 1989), 46.

36. Ibid., 47.

37. Ibid., 25.

38. Ibid., 199.

39. Ibid., 194.

40. Ibid., 197.

41. Ibid., 283.

42. Ibid.

43. Flannery O'Connor, *The Complete Stories* (New York: Harcourt Brace, 1971), 133.

44. Ursula King, *Spirit of Fire: The Life and Vision of Teilhard de Chardin* (Maryknoll, NY: Orbis Books, 1998), 100.

45. Karl Rahner, *Spiritual Writings* (Modern Spiritual Masters Series), ed. by Philip Endean (Maryknoll, NY: Orbis Books, 2004), 24.

46. Cardinal Emmanuel Célistin Suhard, *Priests among Men* (Whitefish, MT: Literary Licensing, 2011).

47. Franz Kafka, from a letter to Max Brod, end of March, 1918 (possibly quoting Kierkegaard, or Brod back to himself), *Letters*

to Friends, Family, and Editors, trans. Richard and Clara Winston (Berlin: Schocken Books, 1977), 203.

48. Thomas R. Cole, Nathan S. Carlin, and Ronald A. Carson, *Medical Humanities: An Introduction* (New York: Cambridge University Press, 2015), 28. See also www.nlm.nih.gov/hmd/greek/greek_oath.html.

49. Franz Kafka, letter to Max Brod, mid-September, 1917, in *Letters to Friends, Family, and Editors*, trans. Richard and Clara Winston (Berlin: Schocken Books, 1977), 138.

50. Ibid.

51. Ibid., 74.

52. Ibid., 3.

53. Ibid., 10.

54. Ibid., 323.

55. Ibid.

56. Ibid., 333.

57. Joseph Cardinal Ratzinger, unpublished homily, March 22, 1978, in Pope Benedict XVI, *Co-Workers of the Truth: Meditations for Every Day of the Year*, ed. Sister Irene Grassl (San Francisco: Ignatius Press, 1992), 359.

58. Susan M. Love, MD, with Karen Lindsey, *Dr. Susan Love's Breast Book* (New York: Perseus Books, 1995), 424.

59. Ralph W. Moss, PhD, *The Cancer Industry* (St. Paul, MN: Paragon House, 1991), 73–74. Dr. Moss was fired in 1977 as assistant director of public affairs at New York's Memorial

Sloan-Kettering Cancer Center for opposing their cover-up of positive research results on Laetrile and has been crusading for alternative treatments ever since. Another of his books I found helpful was *Questioning Chemotherapy.*

60. Susan M. Love, MD, with Karen Lindsey, *Dr. Susan Love's Breast Book* (New York: Perseus Books, 1995), 325, 329.

61. "It is too soon to tell how many women we are curing, if any, but for those we don't cure, it is safe to say that we are prolonging their life span two to three years beyond what they would have had without chemotherapy." Susan M. Love, MD, with Karen Lindsey, *Dr. Susan Love's Breast Book* (New York: Perseus Books, 1995), 325–26.

62. St. John of the Cross, *Ascent of Mount Carmel* (Liguori, MO: Triumph Books, 1991), 58.

63. Caryll Houselander, *Wood of the Cradle, Wood of the Cross: The Little Way of the Infant Jesus* (Manchester, NH: Sophia Institute Press, 1995), 19.

64. Susan M. Love, MD, with Karen Lindsey, *Dr. Susan Love's Breast Book.* (New York: Perseus Books, 1995), 281–82.

65. Ibid., 458–59.

66. Ibid., 323.

67. Derrick Jensen, "Why We Can't Trust the Cancer Establishment: An Interview with Samuel Epstein," *The Sun*, March, 2000, 10. In *The Politics of Cancer* and elsewhere, Epstein argues that behemoths like the National Cancer Institute and the American Cancer Society refuse to admit that most cancers are caused by

environmental toxins because they don't want to antagonize the chemical and pharmaceutical companies that largely *fund* them.

68. Ibid.

69. Susan M. Love, MD, with Karen Lindsey, *Dr. Susan Love's Breast Book* (New York: Perseus Books, 1995), 324.

70. See Michael W. DeGregorio and Valerie J. Wiebe, *Tamoxifen and Breast Cancer: What Everyone Should Know about the Treatment of Breast Cancer* (New Haven, CT: Yale University Press, 1999), 65: "Perhaps one of the most alarming findings in the study of tamoxifen resistance is the evidence in humans and animals that after continued exposure to tamoxifen, tumors may actually become dependent on the drug for growth."

71. John Monczunski, "Prescription for Trouble," *Notre Dame Magazine* 28, no. 4 (winter 1999–2000): 20.

72. Malcolm Gladwell, "John Rock's Error: What the Co-inventor of the Pill Didn't Know: Menstruation Can Endanger Women's Health" *The New Yorker* (March 13, 2000): 52. See also http://gladwell.com/john-rock-s-error/.

73. Elisabeth Leseur, *The Secret Diary of Elisabeth Leseur: The Woman Whose Goodness Changed Her Husband from Atheist to Priest,* (Manchester, NH: Sophia Institute Press, 2002), 129

74. Paul C. Bragg and Patricia Bragg, *The Miracle of Fasting* (Santa Barbara, CA: Health Science, 1994), iii.

75. Ibid., 151.

76. Ibid., 47.

77. Ibid., 32.

78. Ibid., 3.

79. Ibid., 4.

80. Ibid., 19.

81. Ibid.

82. Kenzaburo Oe, *Hiroshima Notes* (New York: Grove Press, 1986), 182.

83. Susan M. Love, MD, with Karen Lindsey, *Dr. Susan Love's Breast Book* (New York: Perseus Books, 1995), 402.

84. Ibid., 412.

85. Ibid.

86. Ibid., 413.

87. Ibid., 414.

88. Several sources corroborated this, among them Steve Austin, ND, and Cathy Hitchcock, MSW, *Breast Cancer: What You Should Know (But May Not Be Told) About Prevention, Diagnosis and Treatment* (New York: Harmony Books, 1994), 49: ("[R]adiation does not improve your chances of surviving breast cancer."); Ralph W. Moss, *The Cancer Industry* (St. Paul, MN: Paragon House, 1991), 62: ("In a 1968 study of 3000 women [being treated for breast cancer] at over 40 institutions, [Dr. Bernard Fisher of the University of Pittsburgh] found that those receiving postoperative radiation did no better than those receiving only surgery in the treatment of breast cancer."); and an AP article entitled "Drop in Breast Cancer Deaths Tied to Treatment," *Los Angeles Times* (May 19, 2000): "Radiation, the oldest [breast cancer] treatment, prevents about two-thirds of recurrences but

has yielded only a 1% decrease in the overall death rates. Although it works well in clearing up rogue bits of cancer in the breast, it also increases the risk of heart attacks and strokes."

89. Jerome Groopman, "The Doubting Disease: When Is Obsession a Sickness?" *The New Yorker* (April 10, 2000): 52. See also www.newyorker.com/archive/2000/04/10/2000_04_10_052_TNY_LIBRY_000020598.

90. Franz Kafka, *Diaries 1910–1923* (Berlin: Schocken Classics,1988), 228.

91. Flannery O'Connor, letter to Cecil Dawkins, dated December 23, 1959, in *The Habit of Being: Letters of Flannery O'Connor* (New York: Vintage Books, 1979), 365.

92. W. H. Auden, "Lullaby," in *Collected Poems: Auden* (New York: Vintage, reprint ed. 1991), 157.

93. *The Practice of the Presence of God: The Complete Works of Brother Lawrence with Notes and Scripture References* (Colorado: Perieco Publishing, 2009), 82.

94. Susan Sontag, *Illness as Metaphor* (New York: Farrar, Straus and Giroux, 1977), 64–65.

95. "[I]t is one thing to be skeptical about the rhetoric that surrounds cancer, another to give support to many uninformed doctors who insist that no significant progress in treatment has been made, and that cancer is not really curable. The bromides of the American cancer establishment, tirelessly hailing the imminent victory over cancer; the professional pessimism of a large number of cancer specialists, talking like battle-weary officers mired down in an interminable colonial war—these are the twin distortions in this military rhetoric about cancer." Ibid., 66–67.

96. Ibid., 83.

97. Ibid., 84.

98. Ibid.

99. Ibid., 85.

100. Carl Edmund Rollyson and Lisa Olson Paddock, *Susan Sontag: The Making of an Icon* (New York: W. W. Norton, 2000), 171.

101. Ibid., 171–72.

102. Ibid., 172.

103. Ibid., 173.

104. Ibid.

105. Ibid.

106. Susan Sontag, *Illness as Metaphor* (New York: Farrar, Straus and Giroux, 1977), 87.

107. Susan Sontag, interview by Chris Lydon, 1992, www.youtube.com/watch?v=7Mmi03G5oV0.

108. Carl Edmund Rollyson and Lisa Olson Paddock, *Susan Sontag: The Making of an Icon* (New York: W. W. Norton, 2000), 172.

109. Ibid., 174.

110. www.centerforchristiannonviolence.org/data/Media/ Pastoral_Letter_Iraq_War.pdf.

111. Jacques Fesch, *Light upon the Scaffold: Prison Letters of Jacques Fesch*, trans. Michael J. O'Connell (St. Meinrad, IN: Abbey Press, 1975), 86–87.

112. Author Anonymous: www.hymnary.org/
text/i_have_decided_to_follow_jesus

113. Flannery O'Connor, "The Church and the Fiction Writer" in
Mystery and Manners: Occasional Prose (New York: Farrar, Straus
and Giroux, 1961), 146.

114. Many people have used the quote, including Annie Dillard, see
http://en.wikiquote.org/wiki/Talk:Annie_Dillard. The original
source is unknown. See also: http://historymedren.about.com/
od/quotes/a/quote_eckhart_2.htm.

115. See Writing Group for the Women's Health Initiative
Investigators (2002). "Risks and Benefits of Estrogen Plus
Progestin in Healthy Postmenopausal Women: Principal Results
from the Women's Health Initiative Randomized Controlled
Trial," *JAMA* 288 (3): 321–33. doi:10.1001/jama.288.3.321.
PMID 12117397
[from Wikipedia entry for Hormone Replacement Therapy
(menopause): http://en.wikipedia.org/wiki/
Hormone_replacement_therapy_(menopause)].

116. See www.uspreventiveservicestaskforce.org/uspstf/uspsbrca.htm.

117. See www.usatoday.com/news/health/
2009-11-16-breast-cancer-mammogram-qanda_N.htm. See also
www.ncbi.nlm.nih.gov/books/NBK36392/.

118. Helen M. Luke, *Dark Wood to White Rose: Journey and
Transformation in Dante's Divine Comedy* (New York, Parabola
Books, 1989), 136.

About the Author

Heather King is a Catholic convert with several books, among them *Parched; Redeemed; Shirt of Flame; Poor Baby;* and *Stumble: Virtue, Vice and the Space Between*. She writes a weekly column on arts and culture for *The Tidings*, lives in Los Angeles, and blogs at Heather-King.com.